Hope in the Face of Challenge

Hope in the Face of Challenge
Innovations in Rural Health Care

By
Thomas D. Rowley

with photography by
D. Brent Miller

Copyright 2004 National Rural Health Association

All rights reserved. No part of this book may be reproduced without permission from the publisher. Permission is granted to reproduce materials in this text if proper credit is given to the author and to the NRHA.

Book design and layout by D. Brent Miller.

ISBN: 0-9755049-0-8

National Rural Health Association
One West Armour Blvd., Suite 203
Kansas City, MO 64111
www.NRHArural.org

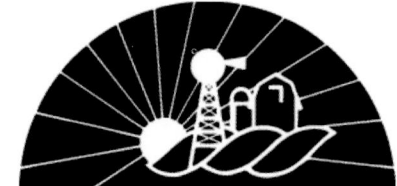

Additional copies may be purchased from:

National Rural Health Association
(816) 756-3140
or on-line at www.NRHArural.org

Payment of $20 per copy must accompany orders to the NRHA and may be made by check, money order, MasterCard, Visa, Discover or American Express. NRHA Publication Order No. PU0804-68.

This publication was funded by the Health Resources and Services Administration, Office of Rural Health Policy through a cooperative agreement.

Foreword

Many are concerned about the state of rural health care in this country, and rightly so. There is great cause for concern. There is also, however, great cause for celebration. Around the country, rural communities are working to meet their health care needs. Unfortunately, their efforts all too often go unnoticed and unheralded.

In the fall of 2003, the National Rural Health Association (NRHA) commissioned writer Thomas D. Rowley and photographer D. Brent Miller to help correct that one-sided view by chronicling the stories of innovative rural health care efforts around the country. The process began by asking NRHA members and others in our network to nominate projects for possible inclusion in such a collection. Not surprisingly, given the wealth of efforts to draw upon, more submissions (all good) came in than could be used. With help from a panel of rural experts from across the nation, the list was culled, categorized, and massaged into the one presented here.

The stories told here are by no means the only ones worth telling. Countless efforts—small and large—are helping rural Americans get (and give) the health care they need and deserve. This book is but a small sampling of those stories. It is, nonetheless, an important endeavor. As Rowley has written elsewhere, "To get its attention, the nation needs to hear stories of rural trouble. To give it a reason to help, the nation also needs to hear stories of rural hope—to be inspired by them, learn from them, and then multiply them."

To inspire, learn, and multiply are the goals of this book and its stories of hope.

Stephen D. Wilhide, MPH, MSW
Executive Director
NRHA

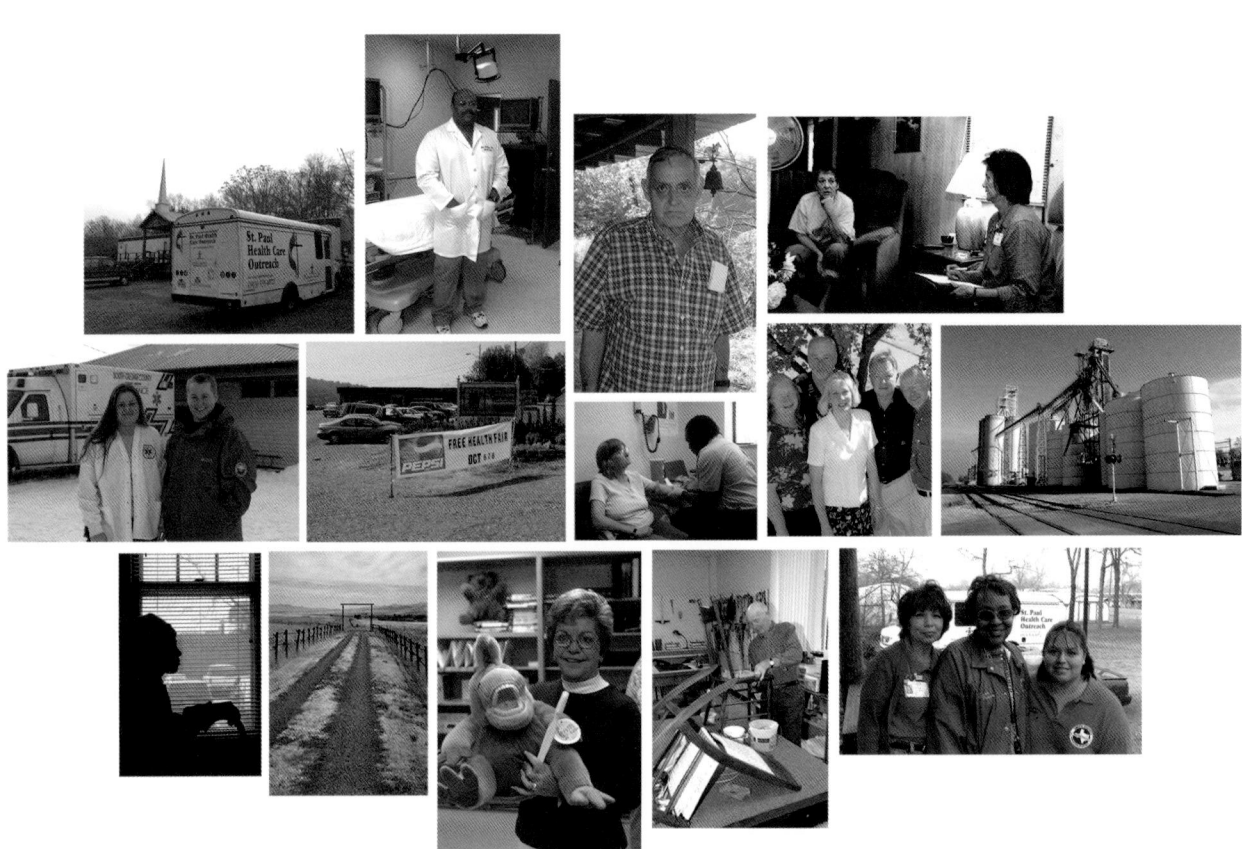

Contents

Foreword by Stephen D. Wilhide, Executive Director, NRHA 5

Letter from Hilda Heady, President, NRHA 9

Introduction 11

Chapter 1–Expanding the Work Force 17
- *Navigating Health Care and More: Southeast Kentucky Community Access Program—Kentucky*
- *Growing Rural Docs: East Tennessee State University Rural Health Fairs—Southern Appalachia*
- *Cross-Training Nurses and Paramedics: Bidirectional Articulation Plan—Kansas*

Chapter 2–Broadening Access to Care 41
- *Rolling Out Care: St. Paul Health Care Outreach Van—Texas*
- *Restoring Smiles: Central California Dental Surgicenter—California*
- *Improving Emergency Care: Comprehensive Advanced Life Support Program—Minnesota*
- *Meeting Mental Health Needs: Sowing the Seeds of Hope—Seven Midwestern States*

Chapter 3–Meeting Special Needs 65
- *Helping the Poor and Uninsured (and Their Doctors): Medical Care Access Coalition—Michigan*
- *Caring for and about Hispanic Immigrants: Wright Medical Center—Iowa*
- *Fighting Diabetes in Kids: Ho-Chunk Nation Youth Fitness Program—Wisconsin*

Chapter 4–Improving Facilities 89
- *Giving Seniors Everything Under the Sun, Under One Roof: Quincy Senior and Family Resource Center—Illinois*
- *Raising Taxes, Raising the Standard of Care: Ashley County Medical Center—Arkansas*
- *Building Hospitals: HUD 242 Program—Colorado and Idaho*

Chapter 5–Reaching the Remote 113
- *Connecting and Supporting Chronically Ill Women: Women to Women—Montana and Surrounding States*
- *Providing (and Paying for) Frontier Care: Gilliam County Medical Center—Oregon*
- *Nursing by Phone: Visiting Nurses of Aroostook—Maine*

Afterword 137

Acknowledgments 139

About the National Rural Health Association 141

About the Authors 143

I take great pride in introducing this inspiring and heartwarming book to you. Thomas D. Rowley and D. Brent Miller have put together an insightful piece that truly captures the heart of rural America and the goodwill of the people who work and live here. The ingenuity of the American spirit is the life-blood of rural America. This book is not only a tribute to the daily lives of rural health professionals and volunteers who have chosen to serve their communities, but it is also a practical tool that outlines the problems that specific rural communities faced, and the solutions that they have found to work best.

As the former CEO of a small rural hospital and the current Executive Director of the West Virginia Rural Health Education Partnerships/West Virginia Area Health Education Centers, I know how difficult it is to provide resources to the rural communities that need them. It takes innovative and creative minds to make the impossible possible, and caring, dedicated volunteers and staff to act on each new idea. The National Rural Health Association (NRHA) believes these innovators are the future of health care in America. While this book celebrates the successes of a few, the NRHA hopes to someday celebrate rural America as *the* success story of American health care. This book is just one of the many tools that the NRHA is providing to help those who are vigilant in the fight for quality health care on the front lines: the frontiers of rural America.

We, at the National Rural Health Association, strive to promote rural health care in America through advocacy, communications, education, and research. Every aspect of our mission is fortified by the voices of people just like you, and the people in each of these stories. We welcome your voice in our common fight for rural health care, and we are proud to raise our voices with you to celebrate these great stories of success.

Hilda Heady
President (2005)
National Rural Health Association

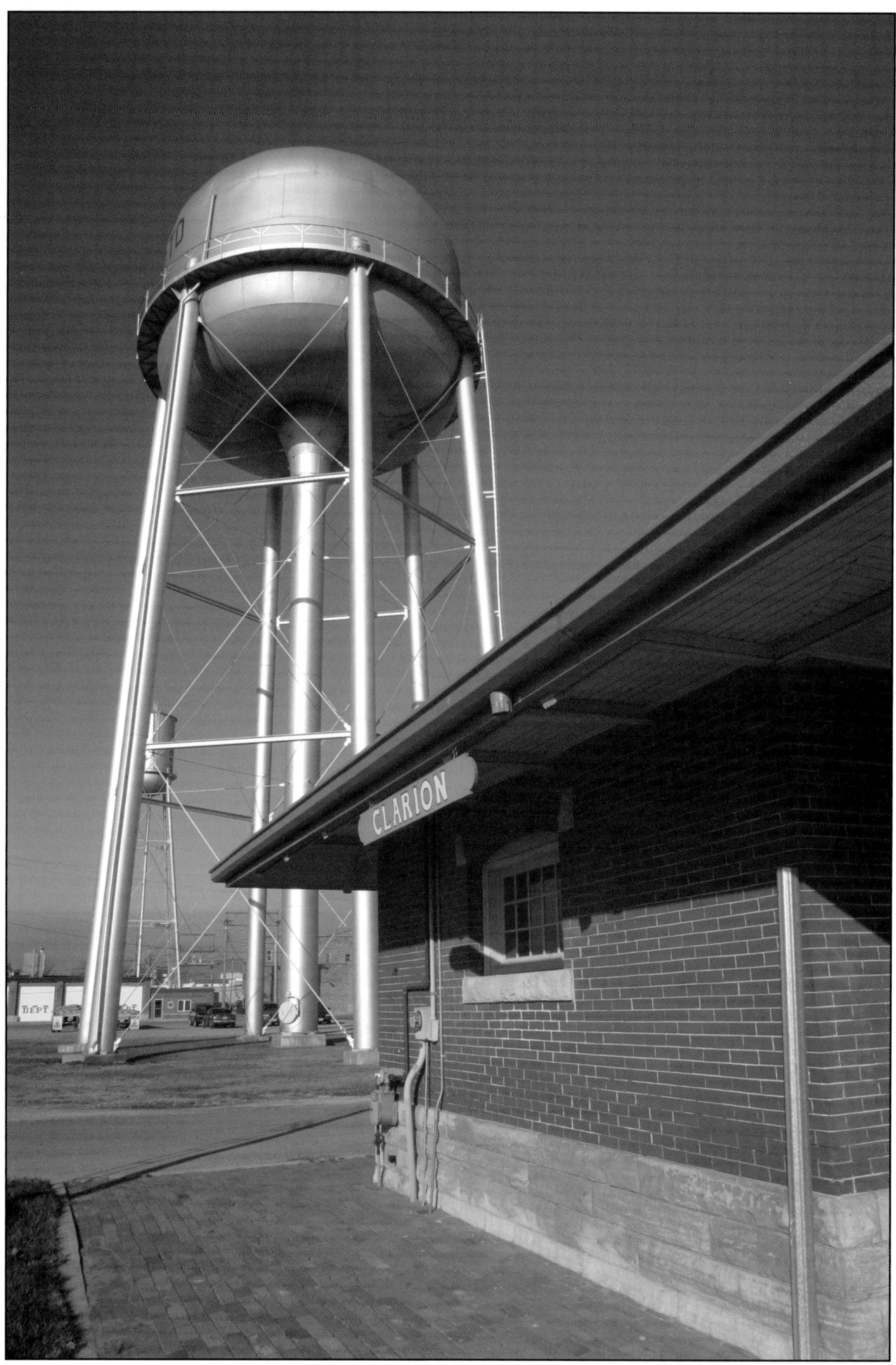

Introduction

When it comes to rural America, often as not, the glass appears half-empty. To put it bluntly, times are tough and they have been for generations. Witness the state of rural health care, or the lack thereof:

- Rural Americans account for some 20 percent of the nation's population yet are served by only 9 percent of the nation's physicians.

- Twenty-two million rural Americans live in Health Professional Shortage Areas or Medically Underserved Areas

- The majority of the 814 so-called "frontier counties" in the United States have two or fewer health care services of any kind. Seventy-eight frontier counties, which are home to nearly a quarter of a million people, have no health care services whatsoever.

- One rural person in 11 has never seen a dentist.

- Nearly three-quarters of counties with 2,500 to 20,000 residents have no psychiatrist; 95 percent lack a child psychologist.

- Rural Americans have the lowest rate of private medical insurance coverage, and one in five have no insurance at all.

- In the 1990s, 186 rural hospitals closed their doors.[1]

Such litanies of statistics, and there are many, are sadly familiar to anyone who follows rural health care. The realities embodied in such statistics are even more familiar to many who live in rural America. Tragically, the "rural problem," as Teddy Roosevelt called it at the dawn of the twentieth century, is alive and well 100 years and countless programs later.

Still, There is Hope

The glass, however, is also half-full. Trite though it may sound, problems truly are opportunities for solutions. In the face of challenge, there is, and can be, hope. This book is about that hope.

In the face of challenge, there is, and can be, hope. This book is about that hope.

Photo opposite page: Clarion, Iowa.

Across the nation, in every state and in every region, citizens and institutions are coming together, rolling up their sleeves, and providing the health care needed to better their lives and better their communities.

Across the nation, in every state and in every region, citizens and institutions are coming together, rolling up their sleeves, and providing the health care needed to better their lives and better their communities. They are doing it with few resources. They are doing it against long odds. But they are doing it.

- In a town of 759 people, miles from nowhere on the plains of eastern Oregon, citizens created a health care tax district (one of the first in the nation) to open and run an around-the-clock health clinic staffed by not one, but two physician assistants, a medical technician, an office manager, and a circuit-riding doctor.

- In the hills and hollows of Appalachia, East Tennessee State University conducts rural health fairs to get medical care to people who often go without and to show medical students the rewards of rural practice so that one day they might become rural doctors.

- In the cornfields of Iowa, the hospital, doctors, social agencies, and citizens see to it that no one goes without needed care. Through the Clarion Free Clinic and the Domestic/Sexual Assault Outreach Center, poor, uninsured immigrants from Central and South America (many without documents) who work in the region's pork and poultry industries receive free medical care, counseling, and support.

- In the remote reaches of Montana and other parts of the West, chronically ill women, miles from health care let alone peers who carry the same burden, are linked together via the Internet in a virtual support group—sharing information, sharing encouragement, sharing themselves.

- In the Upper Peninsula of Michigan, 100 percent of Marquette County's physicians and 40 percent of its dentists have volunteered to provide free care—with dignity—to the poor and uninsured. The doctors and dentists also benefit by seeing the care they provide supplemented with free laboratory work and prescription drugs and by being relieved of the paperwork burden.

- In East Texas, a public health district, a foundation, and local churches partner to provide care through a mobile health clinic to residents—many of them poor and uninsured and who otherwise have no medical care—across an eight-county region.

- In Arkansas, citizens imposed a one-cent sales tax upon themselves to fund construction of a new hospital to replace the dilapidated wood-frame structure built in the 1950s. In turn, the hospital has brought in specialists and increased the availability of services in a county where the next nearest hospital is 45 miles.

- In Kentucky, lay health workers help steer fellow citizens through the health and social services system and help them avoid the many potholes that lie waiting to trip if not swallow them. These Family Health Navigators help clients obtain everything from doctor's appointments and medicines to roof repair—whatever is needed to ensure their well-being.

- In California's Central Valley, young children and developmentally disabled adults for whom traditional dental treatment is problematic, if not impossible, receive comprehensive care under general anesthesia. The clinic serves patients from as far away as 250 miles.

- In Illinois, rural seniors have access not only to medical care, but also to housing, social activities, exercise facilities, a library, and everything else a senior could need—all under one roof. As a result, no one falls through the cracks.

Far more than descriptions of programs and procedures, rules and regulations, this book is about people helping people.

These and other such stories are the heart of this book. Far more than descriptions of programs and procedures, rules and regulations, this book is about people helping people. It is about heartbreaking need and heartwarming responses to those needs.

Unique Efforts, Common Elements

Just as each rural community is unique, so each of these stories is unique—particular people, particular places, particular solutions. Yet each effort shares themes in common with the others.

Innovative. First and foremost, each of the efforts chronicled here is innovative in one way or another. These efforts bring fresh ideas to bear

13

> *Not surprisingly, the best solutions to problems in rural health care come from within the local community....*

on long-standing problems, even if the fresh idea is as simple as "we can fix this, if we try."

Locally grown. Not surprisingly, the best solutions to problems in rural health care come from within the local community, from people who understand the need and the culture, and often from people who themselves have walked in the shoes of those they now seek to help. Intimate knowledge of the context, the culture, the people, and the need does several things to enhance a solution's chances for success: enabling identification of actual needs, knowing who the partners are that can contribute to the effort, and increasing the dignity with which clients are treated and the dignity that they, as a result, feel. All of these contribute to the most important characteristic of locally grown solutions: trust.

Passionate. If one word describes the people behind these efforts, that word is "passionate." What else but passion could explain their single-minded focus in overcoming such seemingly insurmountable challenges? What else but passion could explain their self-sacrifice?

For some, the passion is part and parcel of a religious calling. Many of the innovators share freely about the role of faith in their efforts. For others, the passion stems from knowing all too well what it is like to be in need.

Partnership. From raising barns to getting electricity to providing adequate health care, partnership is essential in rural America. Resources are simply too few and needs are simply too great to go it alone. And because everyone has an interest—personal, economic, or otherwise—in health, potential partners in providing health care are everywhere…. even in rural America.

Holistic. Humans are complex beings. We are physical. We are social. We are economic. We are spiritual. As such, our needs intertwine. The best approaches to care recognize that fact and deal with the whole person; they are, in a word, holistic.

Empowering. People—doctors, dentists, pharmacists, and technicians included—want to help. Often, however, they do not know how. When they do know how, obstacles prevent them from helping. Several of the stories told here exemplify the power of empowering people to help.

They help people to give, and that is every bit as important as helping people to get. Indeed, without one, you cannot have the other.

Gumption. Taking on the formidable challenges in rural health care requires a certain attitude. Call it gumption, that can-do, must-do notion that says if it is to be, it is up to me (us, actually). The people in these stories would not take no for an answer. Instead, they looked the challenges in the eye and made it happen. That's gumption.

Dignity. Health care should not come at the expense of dignity. Many of the people served by the efforts highlighted in this book have nowhere else to turn for care. They are at the mercy of the people helping them. And merciful is what the care providers are, dispensing not only health care, but respect.

Gratitude. One final common element deserves mention. Without exception, each of the efforts in this book shares this: the overwhelming gratitude of the people who are served.

Here are their stories.

If one word describes the people behind these efforts, that word is "passionate."

Notes:
(1) Office of Rural Health Policy, Health Resources and Services Administration, U.S. Department of Health and Human Services; National Rural Health Association; and Frontier Education Center.

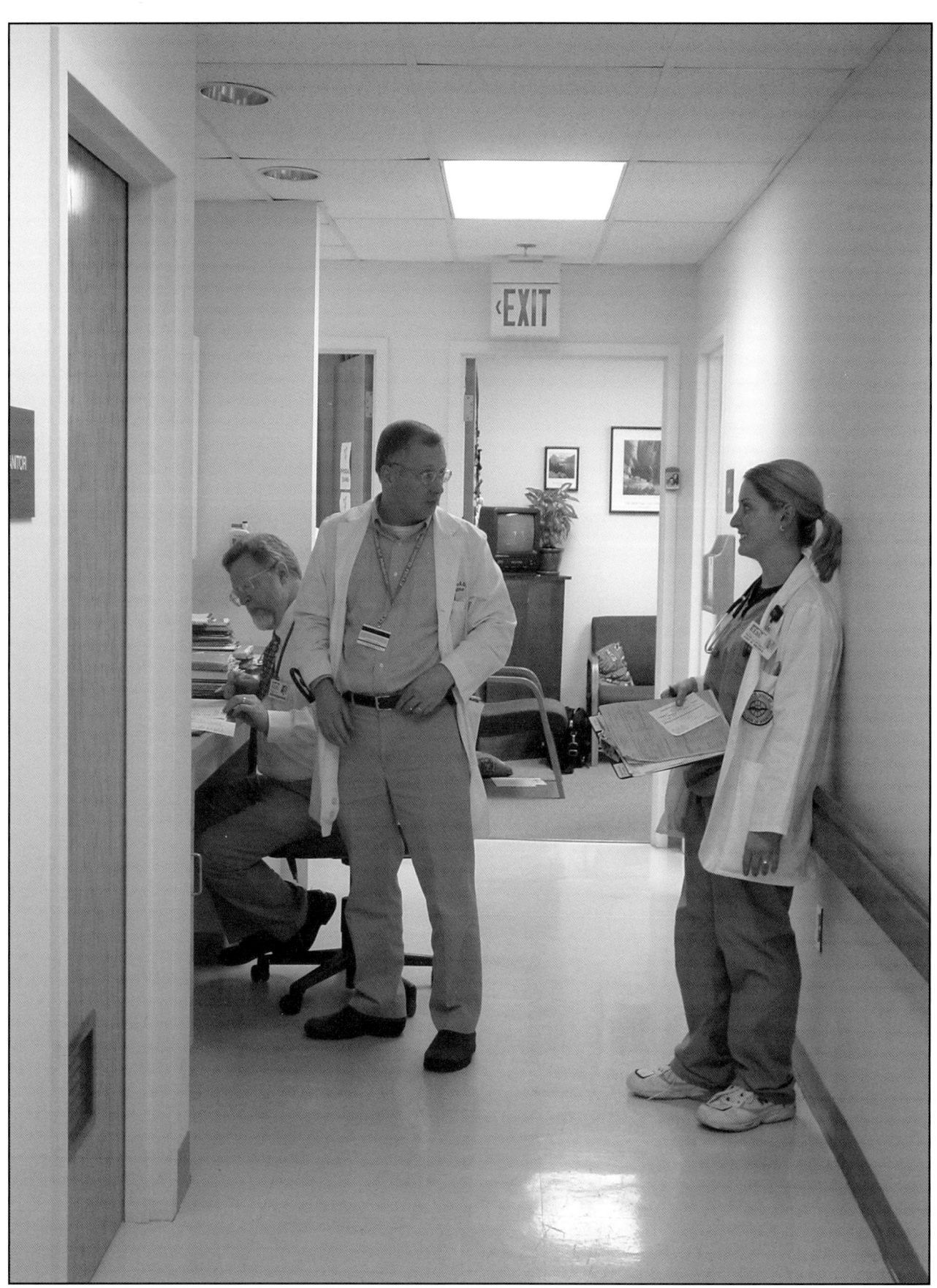

Medical student Amy Brown confers with faculty members Kenneth E. Olive, M.D. and Joseph Florence, M.D. (seated) at an East Tennessee State University rural health fair.

Chapter 1–Expanding the Work Force

The Challenge

Twenty-two million rural Americans live in areas with too few health care providers—Health Professional Shortage Areas or Medically Underserved Areas. Indeed, while rural people account for 20 percent of the nation's population, they are served by just 9 percent of its physicians.[1]

Efforts to recruit physicians and other medical personnel to live and practice in rural America encounter several obstacles: lower salaries than in urban areas, fewer colleagues with whom to work and upon whom to call for help, longer hours and more nights and weekends on call, a lack of urban amenities, and a lack of career opportunities for spouses. Efforts to grow a medical work force meet other obstacles. Chief among these are lower rates of educational attainment and lower wealth and income status, both of which can act as hindrances to entering and completing medical training, and a lack of exposure of rural youth to medical careers.

The Innovations

To expand the rural health work force, communities and institutions around the country are taking new, creative approaches. In coal mine country, the Southeast Kentucky Community Access Program hires and trains local folks as lay health workers. These so-called Family Health Navigators work with underserved clients to get them not only the medical care they need, but also anything else needed to ensure their health, safety, and well-being. From steering them through the maze that is the modern health care system—getting doctor's appointments, tests, and prescription drugs—to helping them maintain a healthy environment at home—repairing leaking roofs, replacing faulty heaters—the Navigators walk alongside clients and help them obtain a better life.

East Tennessee State University takes a different tack. Each year, it conducts rural health fairs in the region's communities. The purpose is twofold: to bring much needed care to people who get too little of it, and to expose third-year medical students to the rewards of rural practice in the hope that one day those students will become rural doctors.

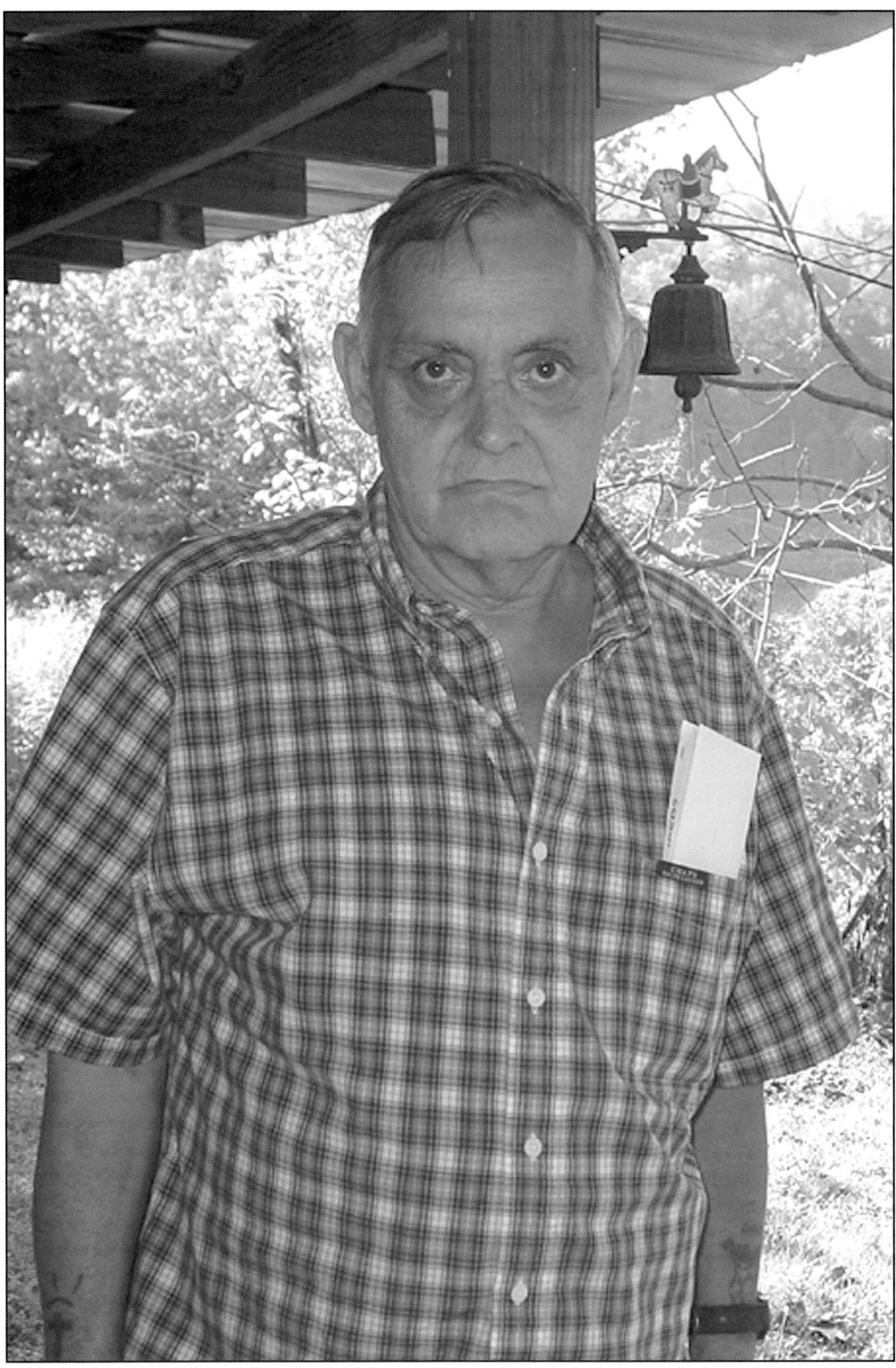

Henry Hall, Hazard, Kentucky

Navigating Health Care and More: Southeast Kentucky Community Access Program

Sabrina Feltner's title is Family Health Navigator, but Henry Hall calls her his "second daughter."

Feltner, 22, is one of ten Navigators employed by the Southeast Kentucky Community Access Program (SKYCAP). Her job: to help folks like Hall, who are uninsured or underinsured, navigate a health care system that is hard to access, hard to understand, and hard to pay for, and steer them clear of the many "potholes" awaiting them.

"Our whole goal is to make them self-sufficient," says Feltner, of the program's clients.

Like most SKYCAP clients, Hall, 56, has several needs. With black lung, heart disease, and a bad back, he is unable to work. Rolling over in bed, he says, makes his heart race, while the pain in his back once led him to drink "two quarts of 100-proof liquor a day," a habit he's since quit. And with no insurance, a daughter in college, and only his wife's department store salary plus the $692 per month he draws for disability, Hall cannot afford the eleven prescription drugs he needs, four of which cost $44 per day.

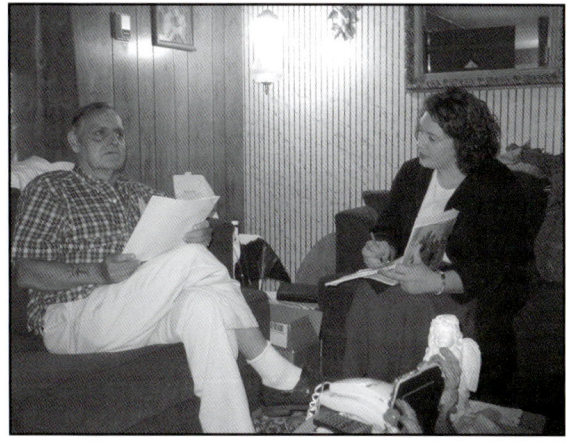

Henry Hall and Family Health Navigator Sabrina Feltner.

"Why, a nickel looks like a wagon wheel to me," says Hall. "I can't come up with $44 just every day."

Fortunately, Feltner helps him get those drugs by filling out application forms for pharmaceutical company free-drug programs, getting him samples from doctors, and, when needed, paying for them out of SKYCAP's emergency medical fund. She does, however, much more.

As part of SKYCAP's holistic approach, she also gets Hall appointments with a mental health provider (whom he refers to as "the nutcracker") to help with his depression, schedules repairs to his trailer (a faulty electric furnace forces him to use a kerosene heater, which aggravates his medical conditions), helps him learn about his medical conditions, and sees to it

> *"Anything I've got a problem with or anything, if she can't help me, she can guide me. I don't know what I'd do without her."*
>
> Henry Hall

that he monitors his blood pressure. Twice a month, she reviews his case with the SKYCAP clinical director to track Hall's progress and to map out the next steps in his plan of care.

"Anything I've got a problem with or anything, if she can't help me, she can guide me," says Hall. "She's come in handy."

As important as anything else she does, however, is the time Feltner spends just sitting and visiting with the man, reassuring him that he will feel better soon.

"When I'm home all day by myself, that helps a lot," says Hall. "I don't know what I'd do without her."

The Program

SKYCAP is one of several lay health-worker programs around the country that employs people from the community to extend the health care and social services systems and ensure that the people most in need do not fall through the cracks. Lay health workers are not medical personnel; they do not perform care or give medical advice. Rather, they educate, facilitate, broker, and navigate. In SKYCAP, the Navigators help clients obtain health care, mental health services, education, housing, and environmental services. In short, they do just about anything needed to help clients manage their medical conditions and improve their overall well-being.

Says Feltner, "We're not a laundry service or a transportation service, but if that's what they need…."

Like its sister program, Kentucky Homeplace, from which it evolved, SKYCAP is administered by the University of Kentucky Center for Rural Health in Hazard, Kentucky. Unlike Homeplace and most other lay health-worker programs, however, SKYCAP adds a case-management component, matching the worker, or Family Health Navigator, with a client for the duration of his or her participation in the program and using custom-made software to enable communication among various providers and agencies to schedule appointments, keep track of services, and chart a client's progress. SKYCAP also has a research component that evaluates the effectiveness of its services.

The SKYCAP program was launched in 2000 with a Community Access Program grant from the Health Resources and Services Administration, U.S. Department of Health and Human Services. The program grew out of two realizations. First, Appalachian Kentucky, like many rural areas, lacks qualified health professionals. Yet getting more doctors and nurses—as desirable as that would be—is not necessarily the answer to the problem at hand. Patients in the region, a large portion of whom have little money or education, need more than what doctors and nurses can typically provide.

As Fran Feltner, B.S.N., who oversees SKYCAP and Homeplace (and who is Sabrina Feltner's mother-in-law, though she neither hired her nor supervises her) puts it, "No matter how many doctors you have, you're not going to get good results without Navigators." The Navigators, she says, complement medical services by filling in where those services leave off. They help complete the continuum of care.

Peggy Caudill, L.P.N., the program's clinical director, talks about what she calls the "ten minutes and ten pieces of paper" syndrome. A patient sees a doctor for ten minutes, is told she has diabetes, is handed ten pieces of paper about it, and told to go manage her disease. Such an experience would be frustrating for anyone. For someone who may be functionally illiterate, may have no insurance, no job, and no money, the experience can be completely overwhelming and of little-to-no help. Navigators come in and pick up where the doctor leaves off.

"The doctor's appointment is just a small amount of health care," says Caudill. "That's just the beginning. People need help understanding the directions—how to take the medicines, how to store them. You don't have time in the doctor's office to do all that."

Second, clients relate best to local people, people who understand their community and their culture; people who, quite often, have themselves needed the services they now provide.

According to Fran Feltner, "A lot of times the best worker is someone who's been on Medicaid, that has had to work the system and had to figure out how to get the services. These [Family Health Navigators] don't take no for an answer. They will find a way … to access the services that these folks need."

Adds Caudill, "There's no 'here comes this foreigner telling me how I

"A lot of times, the best worker is someone who's been on Medicaid, that has had to work the system and had to figure out how to get the services."

Fran Feltner

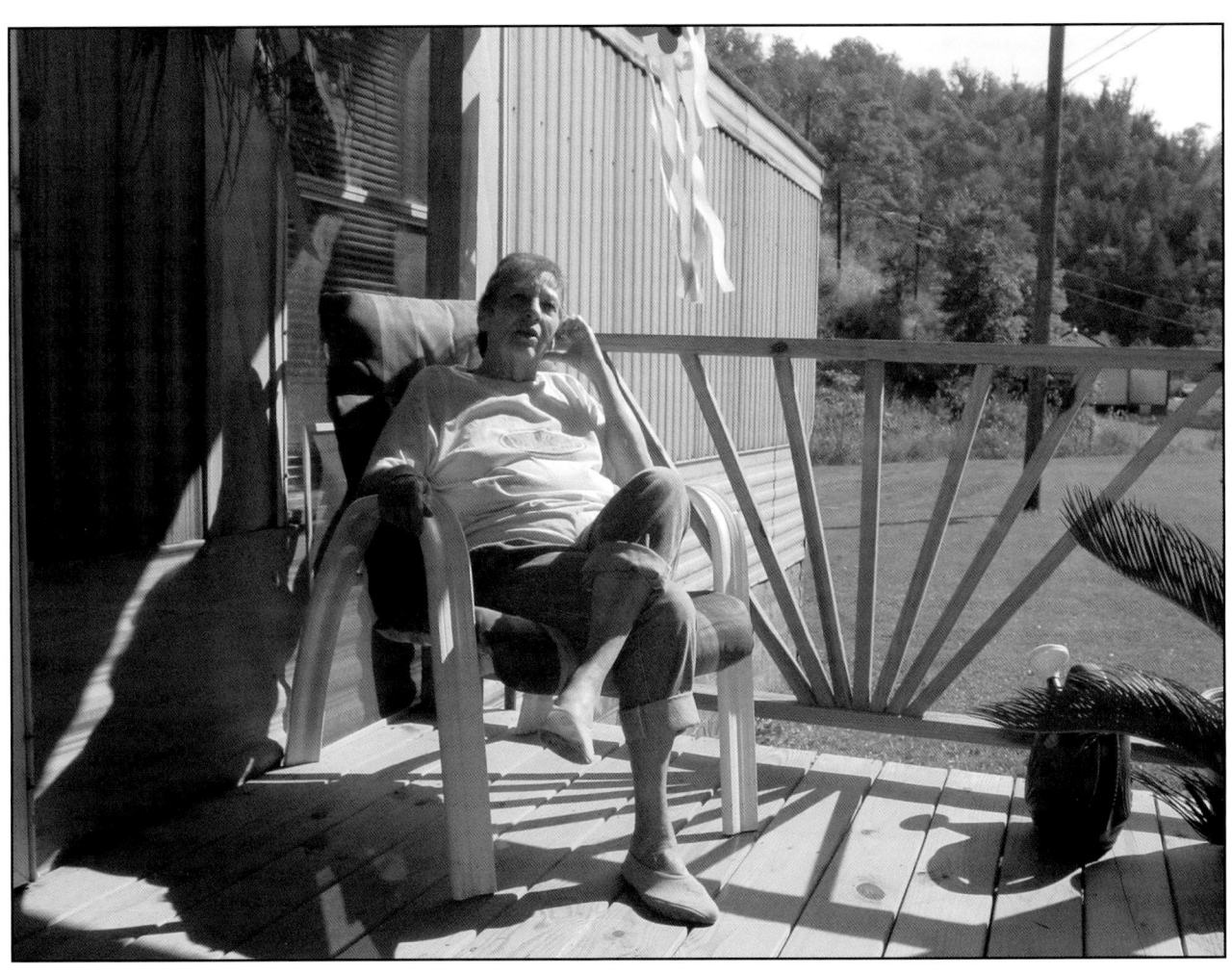

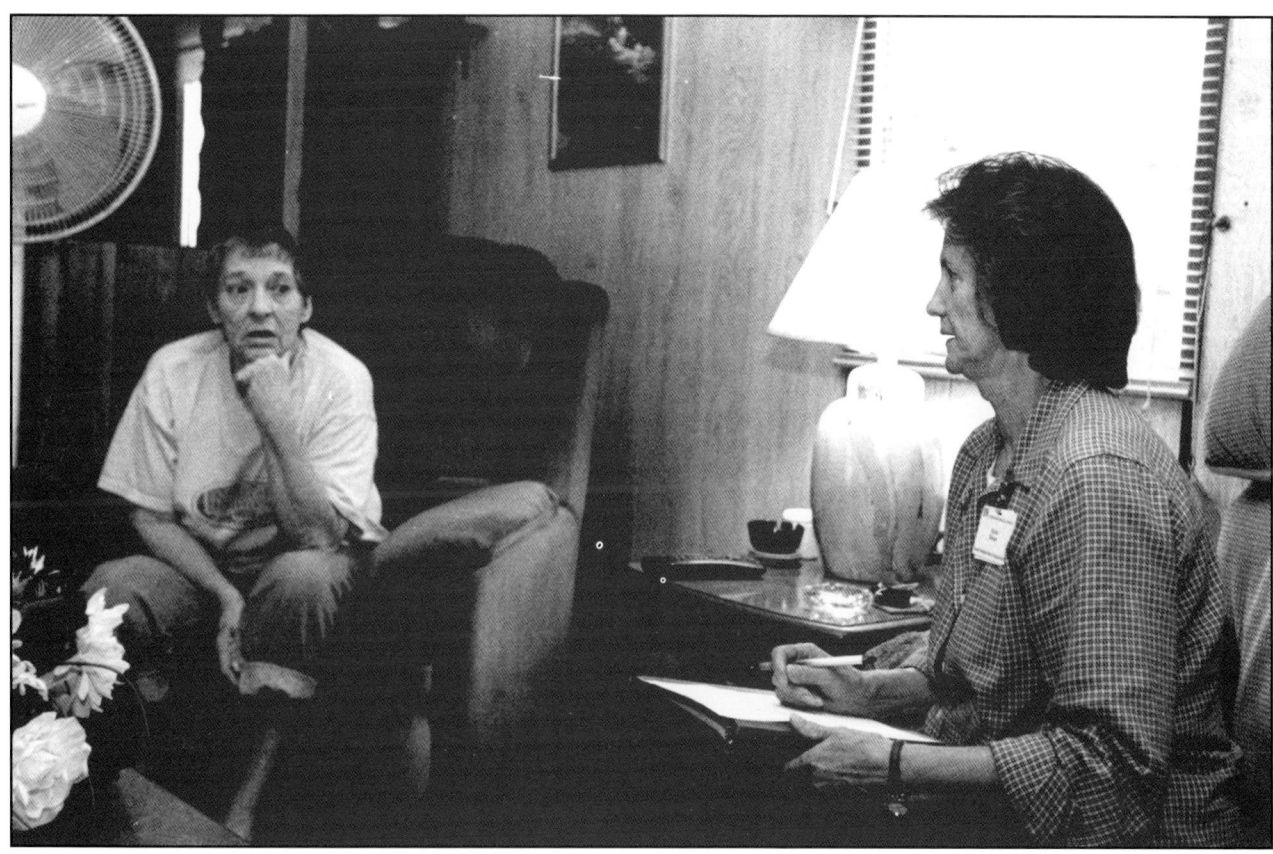

Opposite page: Client Shirley Likens rests on the porch of her mobile home after a visit from Anna Slone.
Above: Likens and Slone discuss Likens' needs.

"We're looking for somebody that's enterprising and that is really dedicated to the idea that you can make this system work for people...."

Judy Jones

need to live my life.' It's the person down the street, so they're automatically accepted."

Sabrina Feltner's experience bears all of that out. Raised in Hazard, she knows the people, knows what it's like to be in need, and knows the system—from both sides. "I can empathize," she says. "I've been there. My family's been there."

In addition to being from the community, Family Health Navigators must have a high school or general equivalency diploma, good communication skills, a knowledge of local services, compassion, and what Judy Jones, J.D., Director of the UK Center for Rural Health, calls an "edge."

"We're looking," says Jones, "for somebody that's enterprising and that is really dedicated to the idea that you can make this system work for people, and not think 'I have a job description that says I do these three things and if it's not one of these three things I'm not going to do it.'"

For such people, the job of Family Health Navigator is a good one; it pays more than $9 an hour in a region where even minimum wage jobs are sometimes hard to come by.

Results

Though only four years old, the program has already yielded impressive results, dramatically reducing the number of emergency room visits and hospitalizations of its clients, saving the health care system more than $1 million, and allowing for a more effective use of the community's resources. It's also been recognized with several awards, including the 2003 Secretary's Innovation in Prevention Award from the U.S. Department of Health and Human Services. Most importantly, the program has improved the health and the lives of its clients.

"I think SKYCAP has had a tremendous impact," says Jennifer Weeber, Director of Community Programs for Community Ministries, one of SKYCAP's founding partners. "I think the disease-management model that we have, using lay health workers who folks trust, complemented with good clinical oversight and good social service oversight, has really made an impact on people and how they view their health."

It helps clients, she says, better understand the preventive steps they can take and signs they should watch out for. "We help folks connect the dots between, for example, their living conditions and their health."

Baretta Casey, M.D., who directs the UK Family Practice Clinic in Hazard and cares for many SKYCAP clients, concurs.

"The program's biggest impact," says Casey, "is the client's increased rate of compliance with doctors' orders, including taking prescribed medicines." The long-term effect, she hopes, will be a decrease in end-stage organ damage, early loss of life, and medical costs.

"I look at SKYCAP as a godsend."

As time runs out in the final year of its federal grant, the program must soon become self-sustaining. One way to do that is to encourage the hospitals, doctors, and other providers to hire the Family Health Navigators. As rationale for such a move, Fran Feltner points out the tremendous costs of uncompensated hospitalization and emergency room visits that providers have avoided courtesy of SKYCAP and the Navigators. One way or another, however, Feltner wants to keep the program going.

"I want it sustained in the community," she says. "I don't want to lose what we've learned. I don't want this community to go back to having no disease management."

"I look at SKYCAP as a godsend."

Baretta R. Casey

Notes
1. Office of Rural Health Policy, Health Resources and Services Administration, U.S. Department of Health and Human Services.

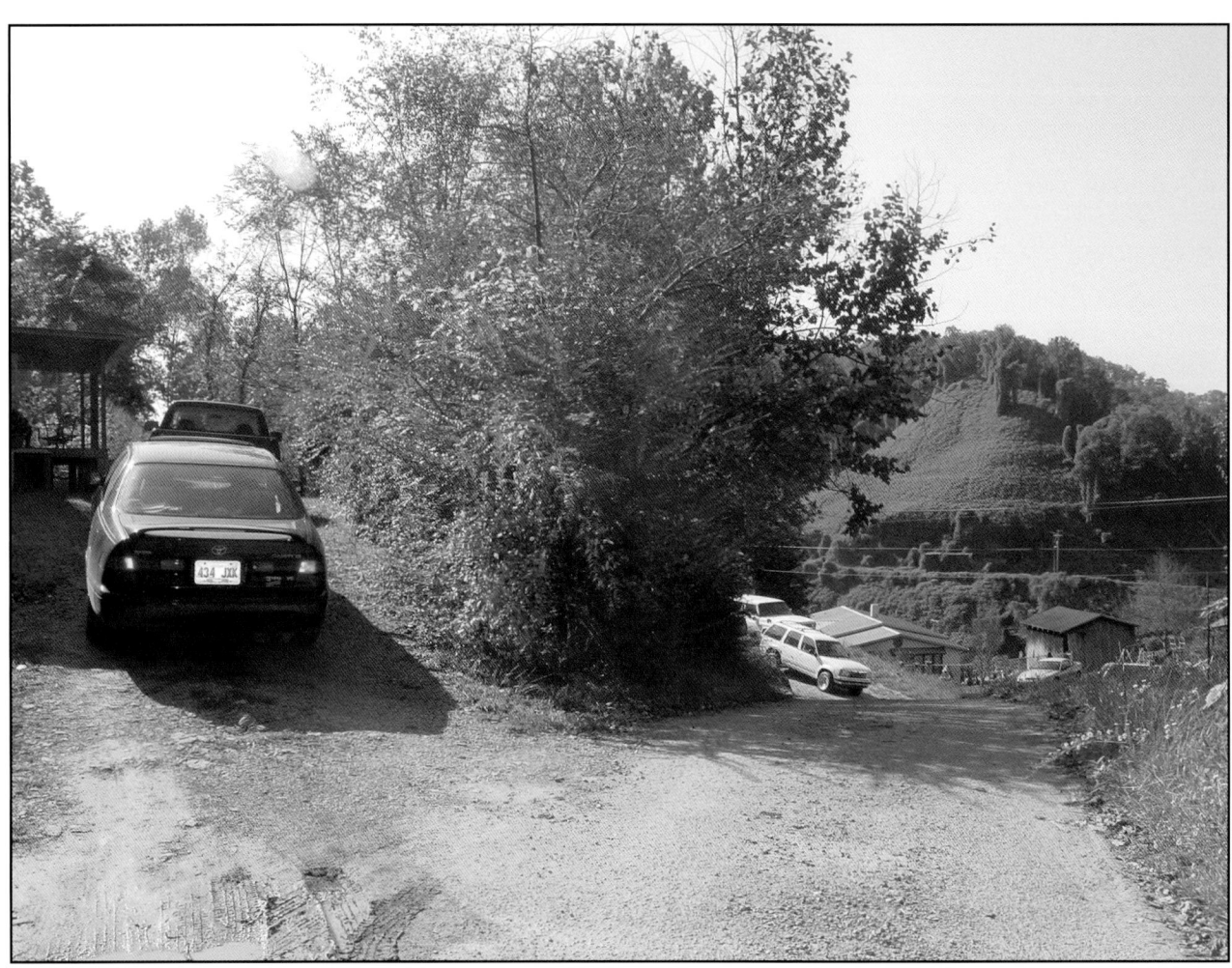

Hazard, Kentucky

Just the Facts

Purpose

SKYCAP uses lay health workers from the community to extend the health care system and ensure that uninsured and underinsured residents get the holistic care they need.

Target Population

Residents of Harlan, Perry, Knott, and Leslie counties in Southeastern Kentucky who are uninsured or underinsured are eligible. Priority goes to people with:
• ambulatory care diseases such as diabetes, heart disease, hypertension, or asthma;
• mental illness;
• housing and/or other problems with their living environments; or
• frequent visits to the hospital or emergency room.

Partners

SKYCAP is a joint effort of the University of Kentucky Center for Rural Health, Harlan Countians for a Healthier Community, Hazard - Perry County Community Ministries, and the Good Samaritan Foundation, Inc., with primary funding from the Health Resources and Services Administration, U.S. Department of Health and Human Services.

Budget

The program's budget was $2.2 million over the four years 2001–2004.

Results

Results to date include:
• more than 10,000 people served;
• 250 to 500 open cases at any one time;
• marked decrease in emergency room visits and hospitalizations, with resulting cost savings of more than $1 million; and
• clients reporting better health outcomes.

For more information, see http://www.mc.uky.edu/ruralhealth/LayHealth/SkyCap.htm or contact Fran Feltner, Program Director, at fjfeltn@uky.edu.

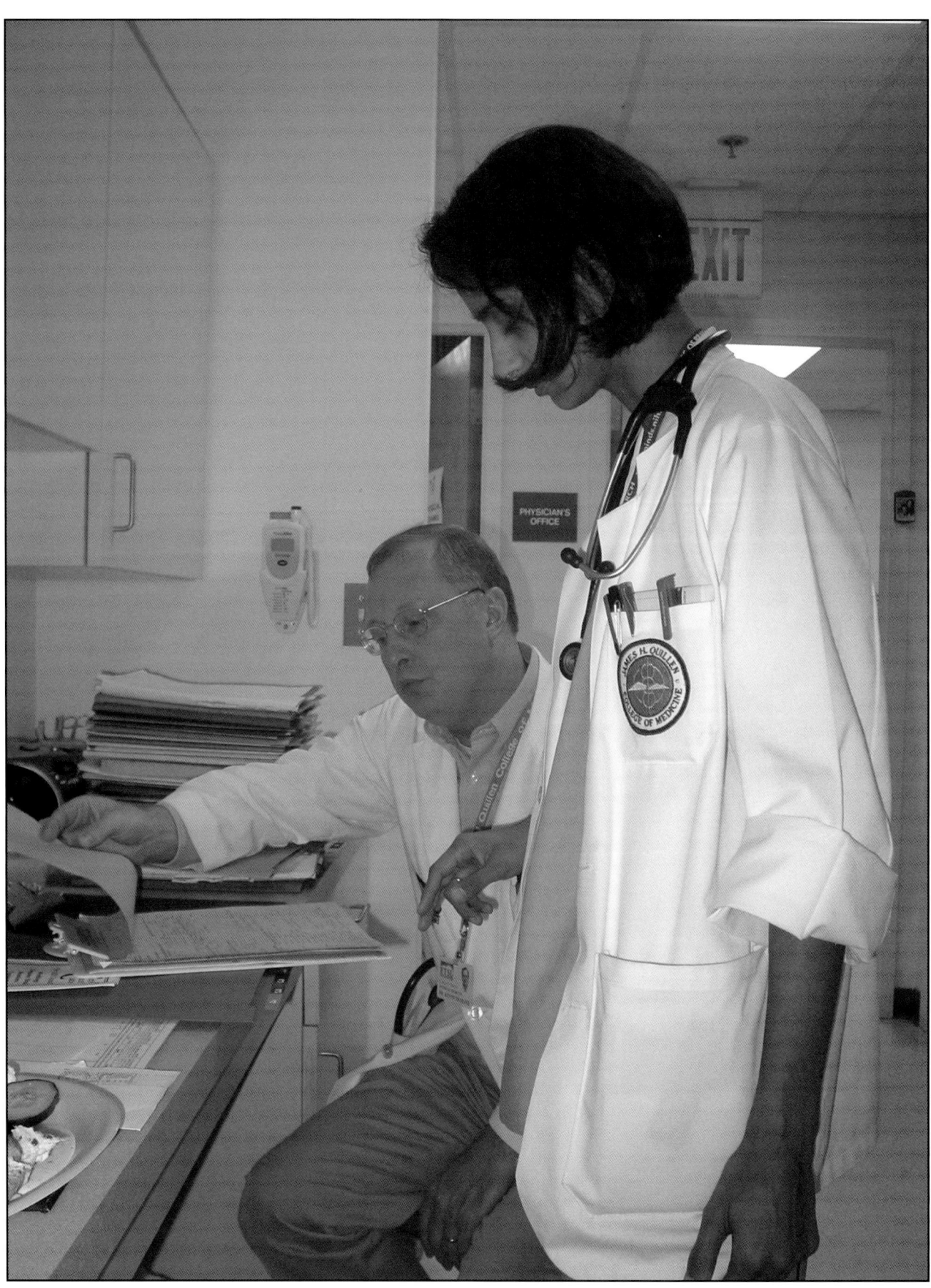
Olive reviews patient charts with medical student Sabrina Shilad.

Growing Rural Docs: East Tennessee State University Rural Health Fairs—Southern Appalachia

The dreadlocks hanging from Dominic Seymore's head mark him as something of an outsider in tiny Saltville, Virginia. His patients today, however, seem not to care.

"You're a pretty good doc," says one man, patting Seymore on the back. Others, mostly older folks, in this Appalachian hamlet are a bit more reserved, if no less appreciative.

"In the suburbs," says Seymore, "it probably wouldn't be the same. Patients might not be as thankful."

Seymore and eight other third-year medical students at East Tennessee State University (ETSU) are in town conducting a three-day rural health fair. Its purpose is twofold: provide care to people who often go without it and, perhaps more importantly in the long run, expose the students to the practice of rural medicine in the hope that they will one day turn into rural doctors, living and working in places like Saltville.

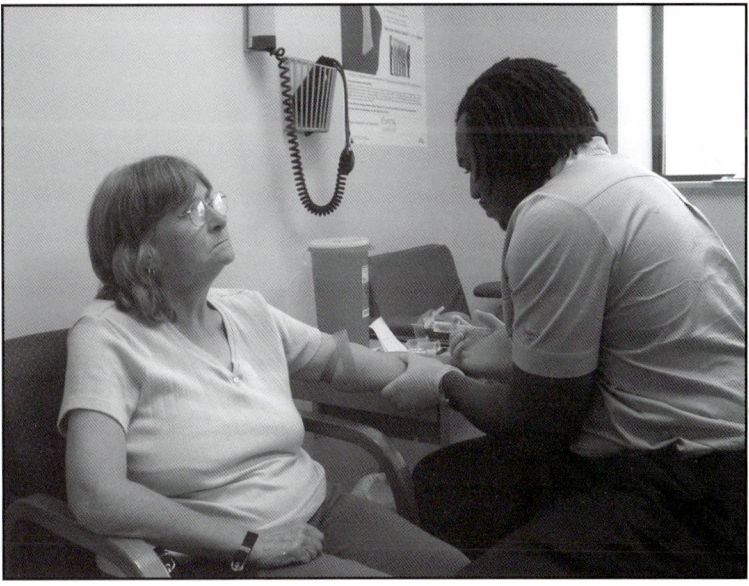

"I think you do the most good in those [inner city and rural] areas and if I don't have a main practice there, I'll do some work in them. I still want to spend time in rural communities."

Dominic Seymore

Drawing blood from Dorothy Everhard, who turns her head so as not to see the needle, Seymore says he's not sure about being a rural doctor. There are, after all, obstacles–less money and greater work load among them. "One doctor for a whole town," he says, "is a pretty busy doctor."

But the health fair experience has had a big effect on the thirty-one-year-old man from Memphis. He's seen how thankful the people have been and he's seen them leave with "a peace of mind." Regardless of his ultimate location, he says that he will help out in rural areas.

"The areas in most need are rural and inner city," says Seymore. "I think

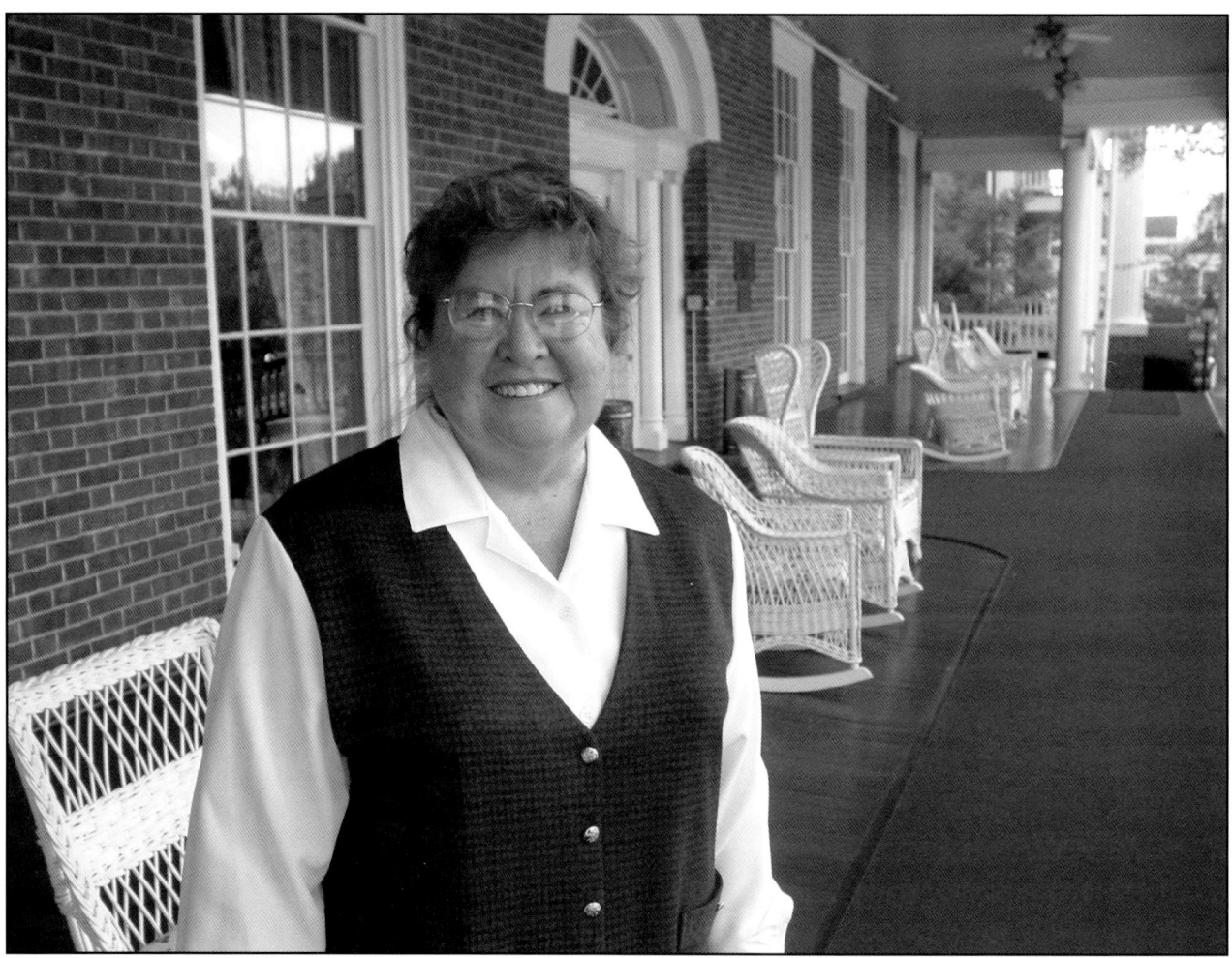
Sister Bernadette Kenny

you do the most good in those areas and if I don't have a main practice there, I'll do some work in them. I still want to spend time in rural communities." Serving those areas and those people, says Seymore, is part of medicine for him.

The Program

ETSU rural health fairs owe their existence in large part to the work of Sister Bernadette Kenny, a nurse practitioner and Medical Missionary of Mary who lives just up the road from Saltville in Clinchco, Virginia. Kenny came from Boston in 1978 and has been providing rural health care—and helping others provide it—ever since. She started out traveling the region and serving people from the back of her Volkswagen. Later, she graduated to a Winnebago-cum-mobile clinic. Along the way, she met up with ETSU doctors and a partnership was born.

"At one point," says Kenny, "the Winnebago would only go in reverse—an apt metaphor for rural health at the time."

Today, rural health in the region is moving forward. ETSU conducts six rural health fairs each year in communities throughout southwestern Virginia, northeastern Tennessee, western North Carolina, and eastern Kentucky. Each fair is a collaborative effort. ETSU provides the students and faculty. A clinic, hospital, school, or doctor's office in the community provides space and some of the laboratory tests. Local churches often get in on the action by cooking for the students while they are in town. Drug companies also provide support of various types. Participation in a fair is mandatory for each of ETSU's sixty third-year students.

Over the course of the three-day clinic, each student examines some ten patients per day. They also see doctors who are excellent role models—doing things they don't have to do, giving back to the community—and interview a local health care provider, asking why a doctor would come to a place like Saltville and what they find fulfilling and rewarding about practicing there.

One of those providers is Jacinto Alvarado, M.D., Medical Director at the Saltville Community Health Center, where the fair is located.

"We help make the students realize that no matter how far away from

Four doctors on staff at the rural hospital where Sister Bernie works are graduates of the rural health fairs. "One went kicking and screaming to the fair."

> *"Students come away from the experience saying 'I really made a difference today.'"*
>
> Kenneth E. Olive

civilization we are, we still practice good medicine," says Alvarado. "It's no different from anywhere else."

According to Joseph Florence, M.D., a family practitioner and director of ETSU's rural programs, the fairs not only give students the feel and flavor of rural life and rural medicine, they also empower the students.

"On campus," says Florence, "third-year students are low men on the totem pole. They don't have the autonomy that they do here. Here, they see the patient, formulate a plan of treatment, and then review it with faculty."

They also learn to communicate with and relate to the people under their care, he says. "It's not unusual, to spend an hour with a patient."

The combination of autonomy and hands-on experience makes an impact, says Kenneth E. Olive, M.D., an ETSU faculty member and primary care internist who, along with Florence, is supervising students at the fair. "Students come away from the experience saying 'I really made a difference today.'"

Bruce Bennard, Ph.D., Director of Faculty Development at ETSU, confirms Olive's observation. In post-fair evaluations, he says, the students express overwhelming support for the fairs. "They see that they can truly make a difference."

And making a difference in patients' lives seems to make a difference in where the students think they may ultimately practice. According to Olive, some even say, "I could see myself practicing in a rural setting."

He knows, however, that the flip side is also true. "Reality is that if you've got somebody who is $125,000 in debt," says Olive, "it's going to be difficult to come practice in a place like Saltville. I'm fairly confident that if they don't have the exposure, they're not likely to become rural doctors."

And helping students become rural doctors is what the fairs are all about.

"We make no bones about saying we think it a good outcome when students choose primary care and go into rural practice," says Olive. "ETSU says this is something we value."

Toward that end, ETSU—ranked third in the nation for rural medicine in

2003 by *U.S. News and World Report*—also runs a whole host of other rural-focused activities: from week-long "growing your own doctor" events for high-schoolers to eight-week rural immersion programs for pre-med college students to its Appalachian Preceptorship Program, which brings twelve medical students from around the country for a four-week stint in rural Appalachia.

According to Carolyn Sliger, M.S.E.H., ETSU's Rural Program Coordinator, the focus on rural medicine is part of the school's mission. "We want to grow doctors that will stay and serve in the region," she says.

The Results

Direct results of the fairs on students' career paths are hard to measure. So many things factor in. Not surprisingly, students at the fair express varying degrees of willingness to serve in rural areas. Some are inclined; others are not; still others are in the middle.

Grant Rohman, aged 24, from Cincinnati, has gained a positive impression of rural medicine through the fair and is open to the idea of rural practice. "This is something I think every medical student should do," he says. "It does make you realize that people in these areas can often go years with untreated diseases. It lets you take a step back and sort of remember why you came to medical school."

Quantifiable results or no, Sister Bernie remains undeterred. Four doctors on staff at Clinchco's Bon Secours, the rural hospital where she now works, are graduates of the rural health fairs. "One," she laughs, "went kicking and screaming to the fair."

Asked if the program works, Kenny replies with a modesty belied by the twinkle in her eye, "I think it does. I hope it does."

"We want to grow doctors that will stay and serve in the region."

Carolyn Sliger

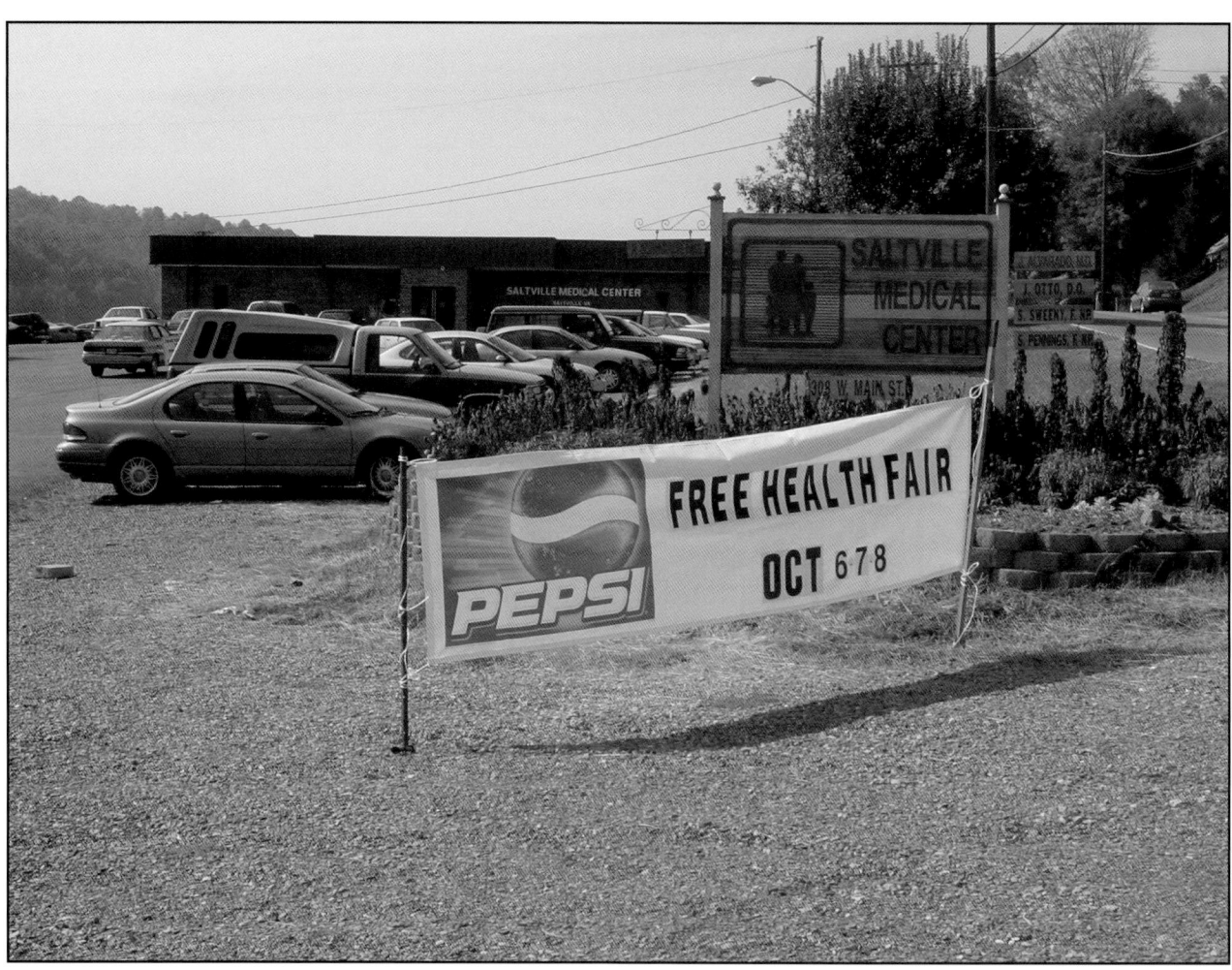

Saltville Medical Center, Saltville, Virginia

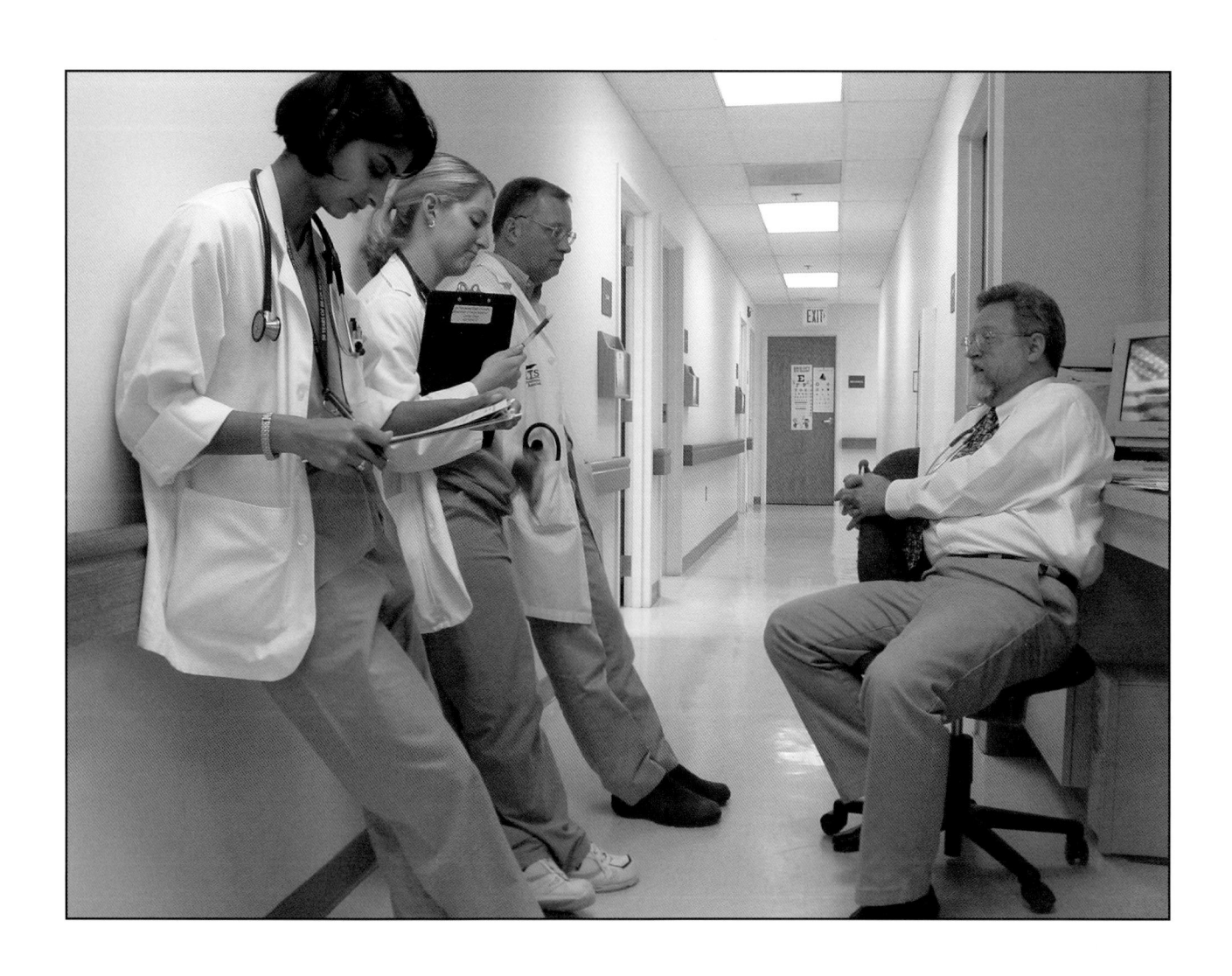

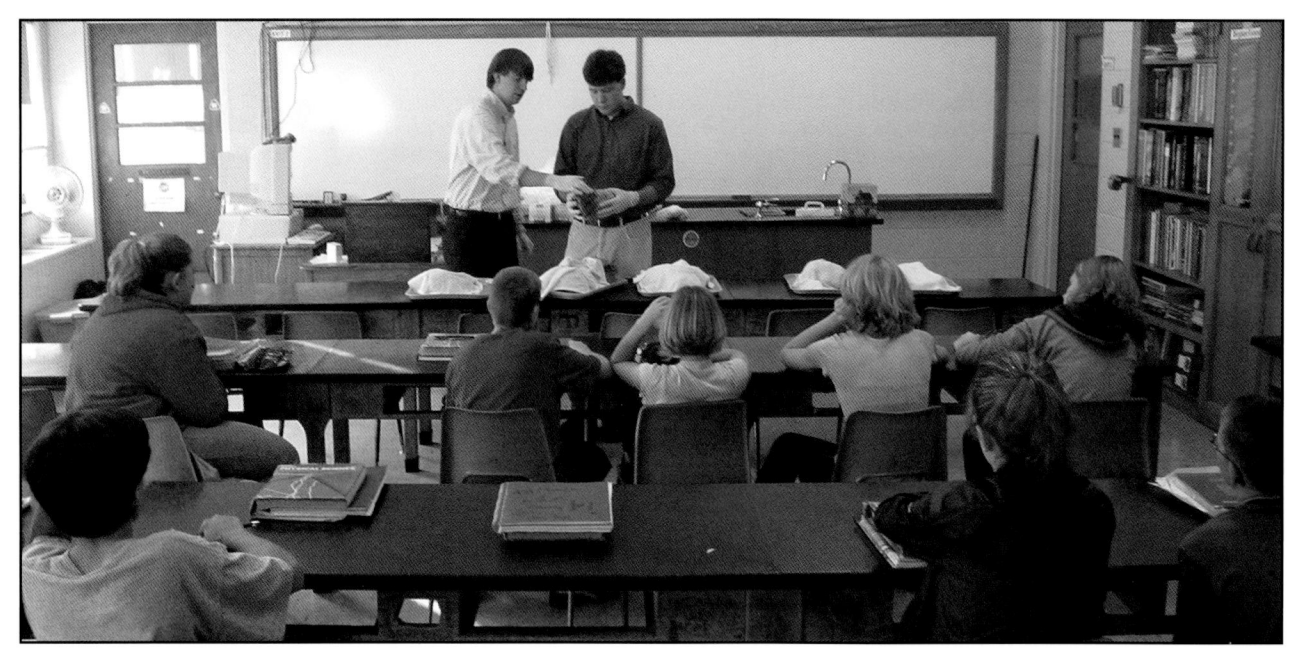

Third-year medical students are often asked to speak to local schools about healthy lifestyles. The 8th-grade class at Northwood Middle School, near Saltville, listened to the soon-to-be-doctors about the effects of disease and smoking on human organs while looking at human hearts, livers, and lungs. The responses from the class were two: "Eeewww," and "Can I touch it?"

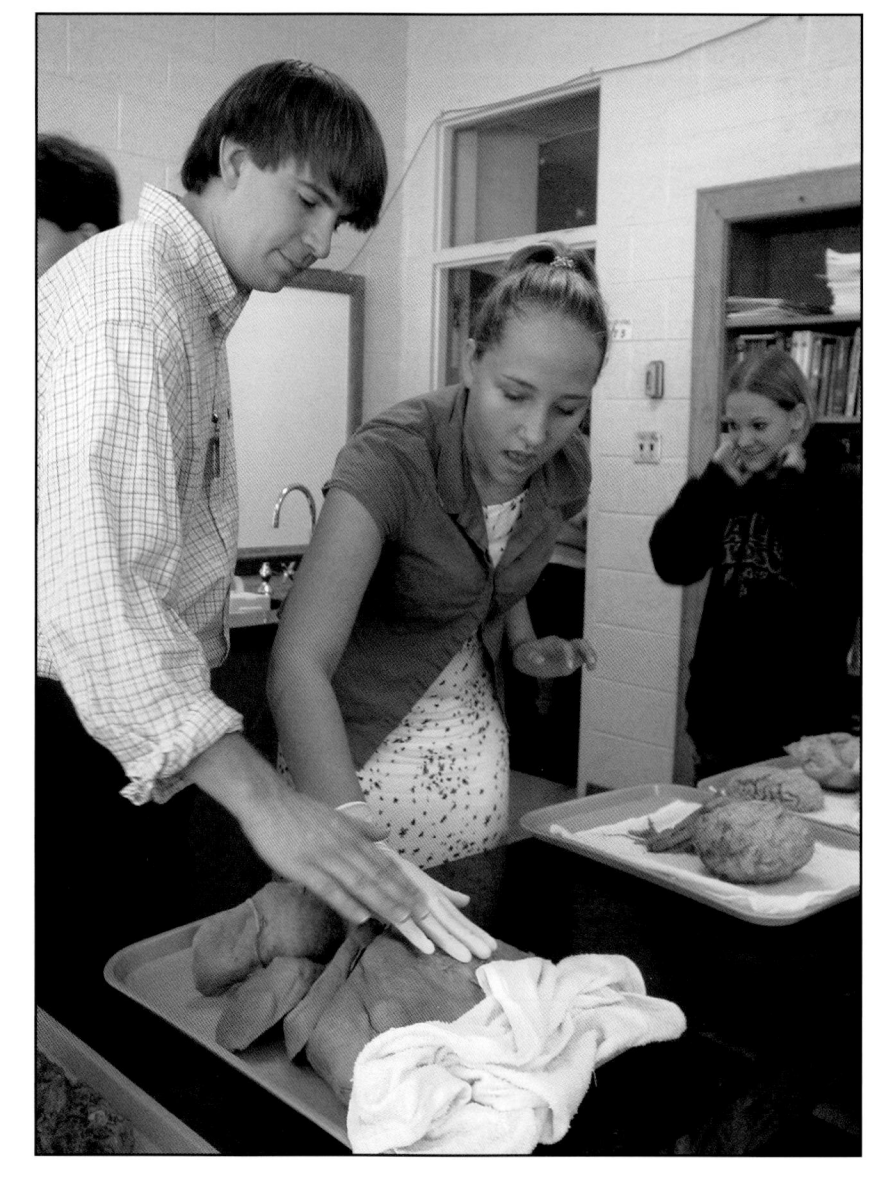

Just the Facts

Purpose

The rural health fairs provide medical students with a hands-on, clinical experience in rural areas to introduce them to the possibilities of practicing rural medicine. At the same time, the fairs provide rural, underserved people with health care.

Target Population

Sixty third-year medical students each year at ETSU participate in the rural health fairs.

Partners

The fairs are a collaborative effort of ETSU; local communities and their clinics, doctors, hospitals, and civic organizations; and drug companies. Funding comes from a training grant from the Bureau of Health Professions, Health Resource and Services Administration, U.S. Department of Health and Human Services, and local community support.

Budget

Each fair costs approximately $3,000 plus the time donated by participants.

Results

To date, 290 students have participated in the rural health fairs and more than 8,000 patients have been served through them.

For more information, contact Carolyn Sliger, Rural Program Coordinator, at sliger@mail.etsu.edu.

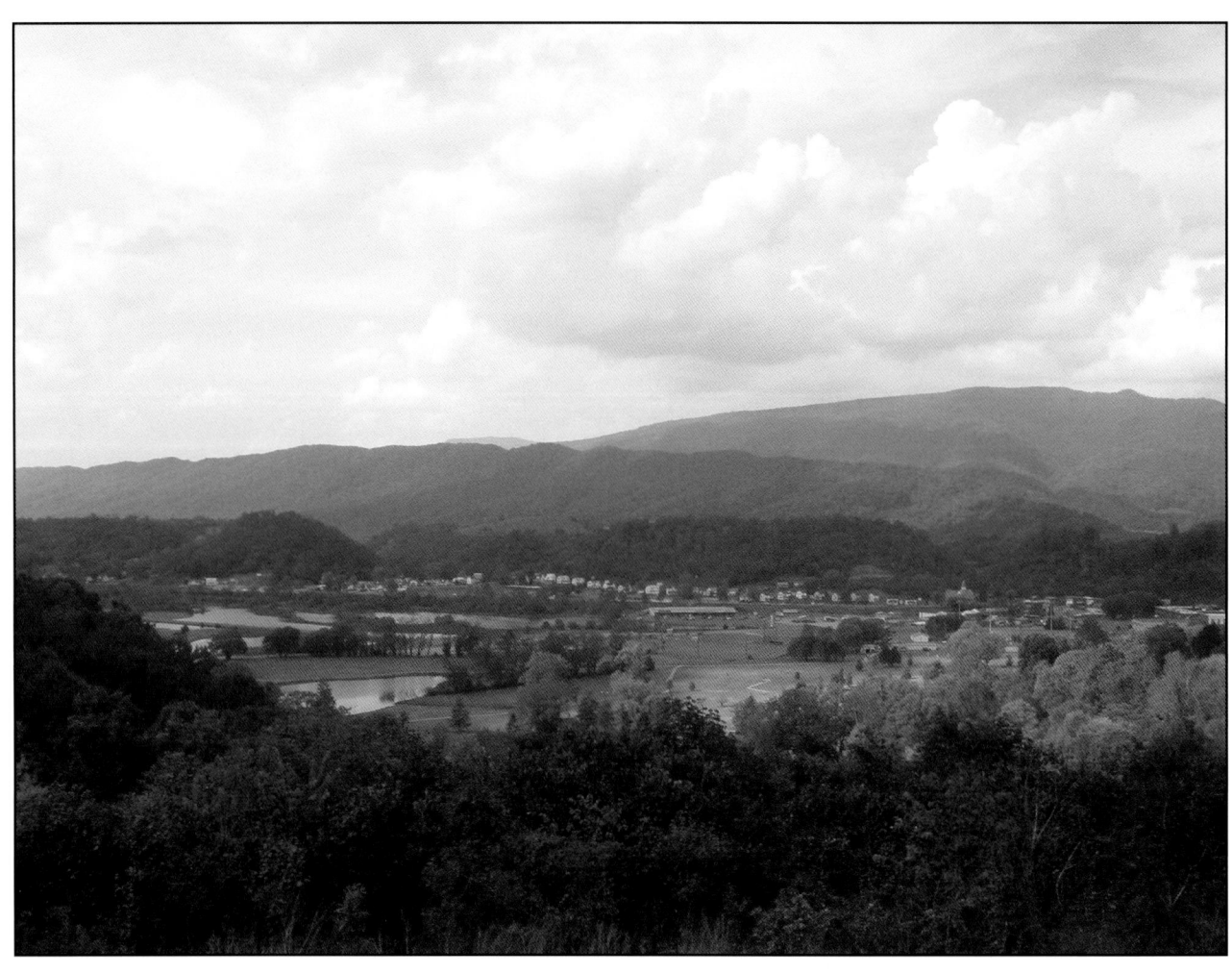

Saltville, Virginia

Cross-Training Nurses and Paramedics: Bidirectional Articulation Plan—Kansas

Working together, the Kansas board of emergency medical services and board of nursing—with support from the state's medical society, hospital association, board of regents of higher education, and office of rural and local health—have created a "bidirectional articulation plan," which paves the way for registered nurses to become paramedics and paramedics to become nurses.

The new plan shows how nursing and paramedic programs in the state's universities and community colleges can "articulate" to allow graduates of one program to enter the other program with minimal loss of academic credit and minimal duplication of learning. In short, it allows members of each profession to bridge into the other.

According to Don White, Deputy Administrator of the Kansas Board of Emergency Medical Services, the plan is based on extensive study of nursing and paramedic training curricula and shows what skills and training a paramedic is missing from being a nurse, and vice versa. It then shows where a paramedic/nurse could be placed in a nursing/paramedic training program.

Whether or not a nursing or paramedic program chooses to use the plan is up to each individual program. Says White, "We've done the work for the locals if they want to do an articulation program."

As in many states, rural areas in Kansas have a shortage of both nurses and paramedics. In response to the shortage, state officials have developed an innovative plan to increase the supply of both.

He also notes that the program is not focused per se on rural areas, but that it would naturally benefit rural areas. Furthermore, he notes that, "By definition, Kansas is a rural state and most of these programs would be considered rural."

To date, twenty nursing programs in the state have expressed interest in pursuing the idea. At least one will begin offering it in January 2005. Similarly, four of the state's eight paramedic programs have expressed interest.

For a copy of the articulation plan, go to http://www.ksbems.org/PRNAK%20Report%202003.pdf.

For more information, contact Don White, Deputy Administrator, at (785) 296-7296.

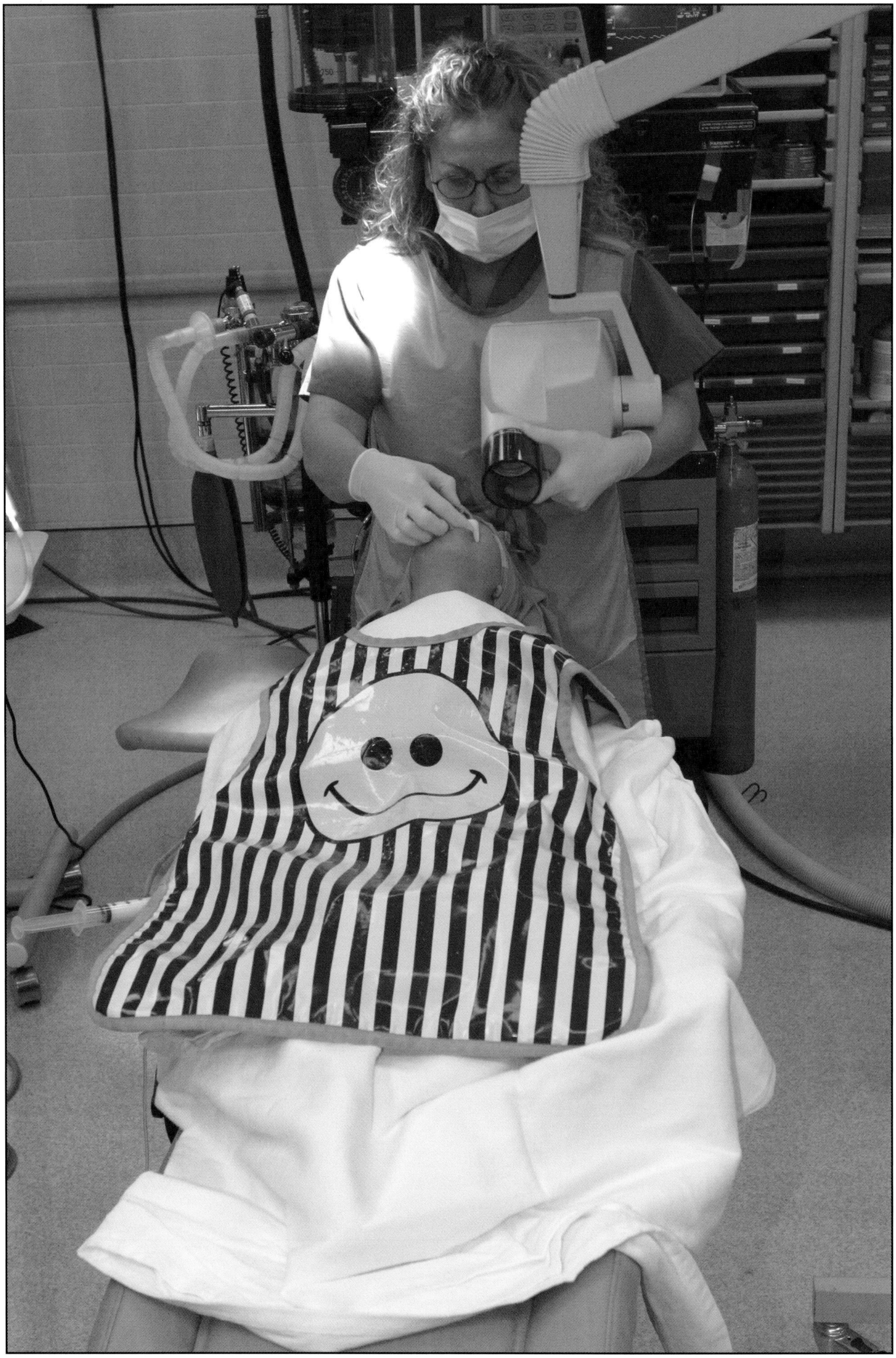

Chapter 2–Broadening Access to Care

The Challenge

Access to care is something of a relative and relatively ill-defined concept, one that changes over time. Just what constitutes acceptable access to care for rural residents? One doctor in town? A hospital an hour away? What about access to practices and technologies that may be called specialties, but because of their life-saving capabilities cannot be called luxuries?

As with other challenges to rural health care, acceptable access to care—in terms of the travel time, a comprehensive range of services, and even affordability—is hampered by the very characteristics that make a rural place rural. Distance, relatively small and scattered populations, and economies that produce fewer high-paying jobs, all limit access to care. As a result, rural residents have significantly lower access to care than do urban and suburban residents, by almost any measure.

The Innovations

Broadening access to care can be achieved in any number of ways. Telemedicine is certainly one way to bring care to rural areas. So, too, is the old-fashioned idea of circuit riding (albeit updated with modern technology).

Residents of small communities in East Texas, many of them poor, are getting their access to care broadened by the St. Paul Health Care Outreach Van. The van brings a mobile clinic once a month to communities in an eight-county region. For most of the clinic's patients, that represents their only real access to health care. Many residents have neither money nor transportation nor even sick leave to travel to the doctor, hospital, or free clinic in the region's big city.

In California's Central Valley, a largely agricultural region, broadening access means providing dental care to patients who cannot benefit from traditional treatment: young children and developmentally disabled adults. In this effort, broadening access correlates to extending the range of services and the range of those served beyond the traditional, more-narrow scope of access to health care.

Photo opposite page: Central California Dental Surgicenter.

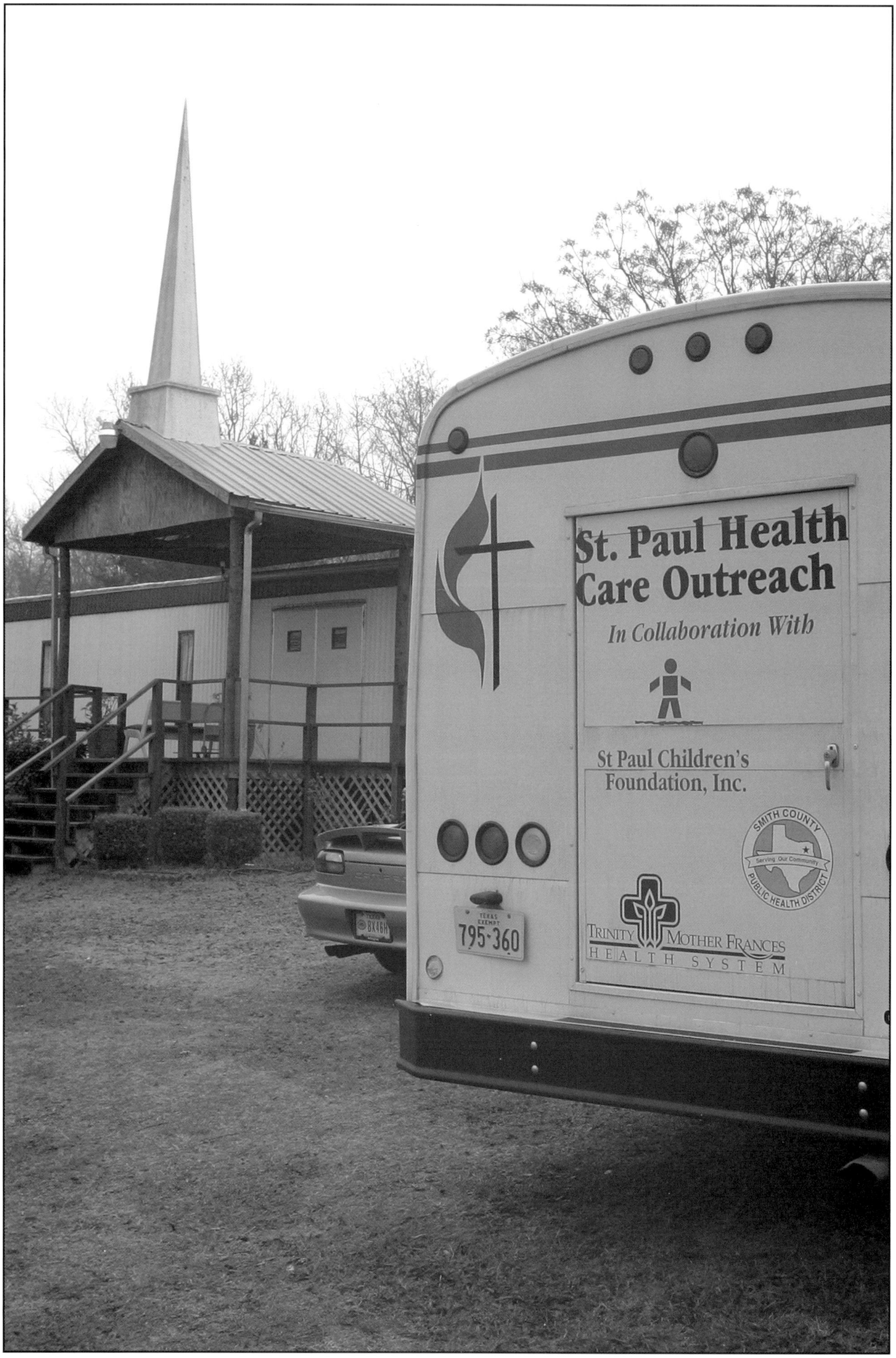
St. Paul Health
Care Outreach
In Collaboration With
St Paul Children's
Foundation, Inc.
SMITH COUNTY
Serving Our Community
PUBLIC HEALTH DISTRICT
TRINITY MOTHER FRANCES
HEALTH SYSTEM
TEXAS
EXEMPT
795-360

Rolling Out Care:
St. Paul Health Care Outreach Van—Texas

Iglesia Bautista del Pueblo sits on a patch of gravel hard by Texas Highway 79, across from a shuttered tamale stand in what might be called downtown....if New Summerfield had one. The church—a trailer with sanctuary at one end, office at the other, and restrooms in between—brings *la palabra de Dios* to the town's large and largely undocumented Hispanic population. Once a month, it also brings medical care to those same people, people who would otherwise have none.

Church member Juan Cabrera sees the effort as part and parcel of the church's ministry. "To help out the community, to bring them closer to Christ, to expand the word of God through this clinic," he says, "it helps us with that."

The clinic Cabrera refers to is the St. Paul Health Care Outreach Van—a circuit-riding health unit providing care in underserved communities in an eight-county swath of rural east Texas. Here in New Summerfield, the van primarily serves people from Mexico, Guatemala, and Honduras who came for minimum-wage, seasonal jobs in the area's plant nurseries. And while the distances the van travels are not that far, at least not by Texas standards (Tyler, the van's home base, is only 28 miles away), the chasms it bridges are enormous.

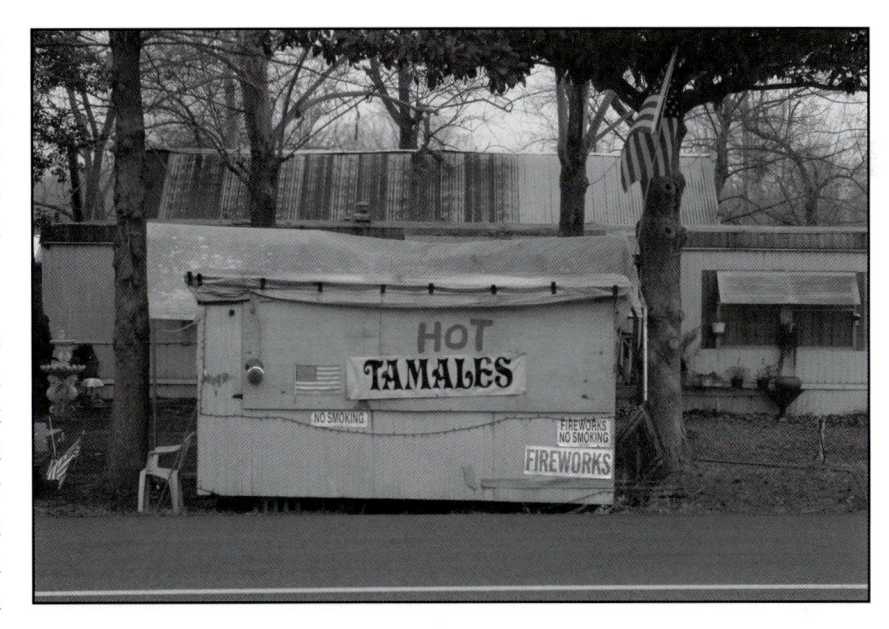

"Without this clinic, the people here don't have any help," says Maria Armas, another church member and local coordinator for the van. "The

Photo opposite page: Iglesia Bautista del Pueblo, New Summerfield, Texas.

> *"They absolutely have mission hearts and mission hands. They see a need, they act upon it."*
>
> Karolyn Davis

people work seven days a week. Their bosses won't give them time off to see a doctor, and even if they do, they have to pay somebody to take them to Tyler." As a result, she says, many would go untreated.

LaJuan Scott of the Texas Department of Health echoes the sentiment. "This project just impresses me so much. It's going out where the people are. If it didn't come here, there would be nothing for them because these are people who don't have insurance. A lot of them don't have the transportation to get into the cities, and even if they did there wouldn't be anywhere for them to go where they could receive the services. It's meeting them where they are."

The Program

The importance and expanse of the effort belies its humble beginnings.

One Sunday morning in 1990, a small Hispanic boy rode his bicycle past Tyler's St. Paul's United Methodist Church, a mostly White congregation of some 100 souls surrounded by a mostly Hispanic neighborhood. He asked a woman heading into the sanctuary if anyone could go to church there or if it was just for "rich White ladies." Heartbroken, Dana Malloy assured him that the church was open to all, invited him to come in to Sunday School, and watched as he rode off anyway.

Fueled by that encounter, Malloy and others she recruited began reaching out to the neighboring community, first by providing after-school activities for kids, then a few years later by opening a food pantry, a clothes closet, and then a health and dental clinic in partnership with the Northeast Texas Public Health District.

Asked how a congregation of so few could do so much, Karolyn Davis, Executive Director of St. Paul Children's Foundation (the organization established to oversee the outreach activities), replies "They absolutely have mission hearts and hands. They see a need, they act upon it."

Fortunately, so did a handful of state legislators who came to Tyler for a tour of St. Paul's health and dental clinic. The legislators were duly impressed with what they saw and asked how it could be expanded to other areas. It so happened that St. Paul had begun planning for a mobile clinic based on a similar one in Houston. However, neither the foundation nor the health district had the money to fund it. The legislature did. With a grant from the state, the St. Paul Health Care Outreach Van made its first run in October 2000.

Like the clinic in Tyler, the van is a partnership between the foundation, the health district, and the state of Texas, plus churches in the communities the van serves. In addition, local governments and private foundations contribute funding or support and pharmaceutical companies supply some free prescription drugs.

Davis calls the arrangement between St. Paul and the health district a unique partnership. "I don't think you see faith-based organizations working with county health. And it works. It's a wonderful thing we're able to do for the community."

"We do everything with partners," says Nick Sciarrini, Director of Northeast Texas Public Health District. "The health district can't do everything we do without partners."

Of particular importance is participation by each of the eight communities. Indeed, the desire to create buy-in and a presence in each location led to the purchase of a small van to merely transport the clinic rather than be the clinic. The van carries health district personnel—a doctor, two nurses, and two bilingual clerks—and some equipment. Examination tables and other equipment stay at each site. Patients are seen in the churches, where, as Davis puts it, "Sunday School rooms become exam rooms and fellowship halls become waiting areas."

"If we're trying to build something in the community and we come, drop the gang plank, go out, flurry around a little bit, raise the gangplank and leave, have we really accomplished anything in the community? We're still the people from Tyler. This way it's more," says Sciarrini.

In that vein, a local volunteer, like Armas, acts as the site coordinator, letting people know when the van is coming and booking appointments for that day. The job, says Armas, requires the ability to say "no."

"I wish we had more [appointment slots]," she says, "because people get sick everyday. People stop me around town, they call me, they come to my house, because I have the appointment book." And the appointment book fills up fast.

"Sunday School rooms become exam rooms and fellowship halls become waiting areas."

Karolyn Davis

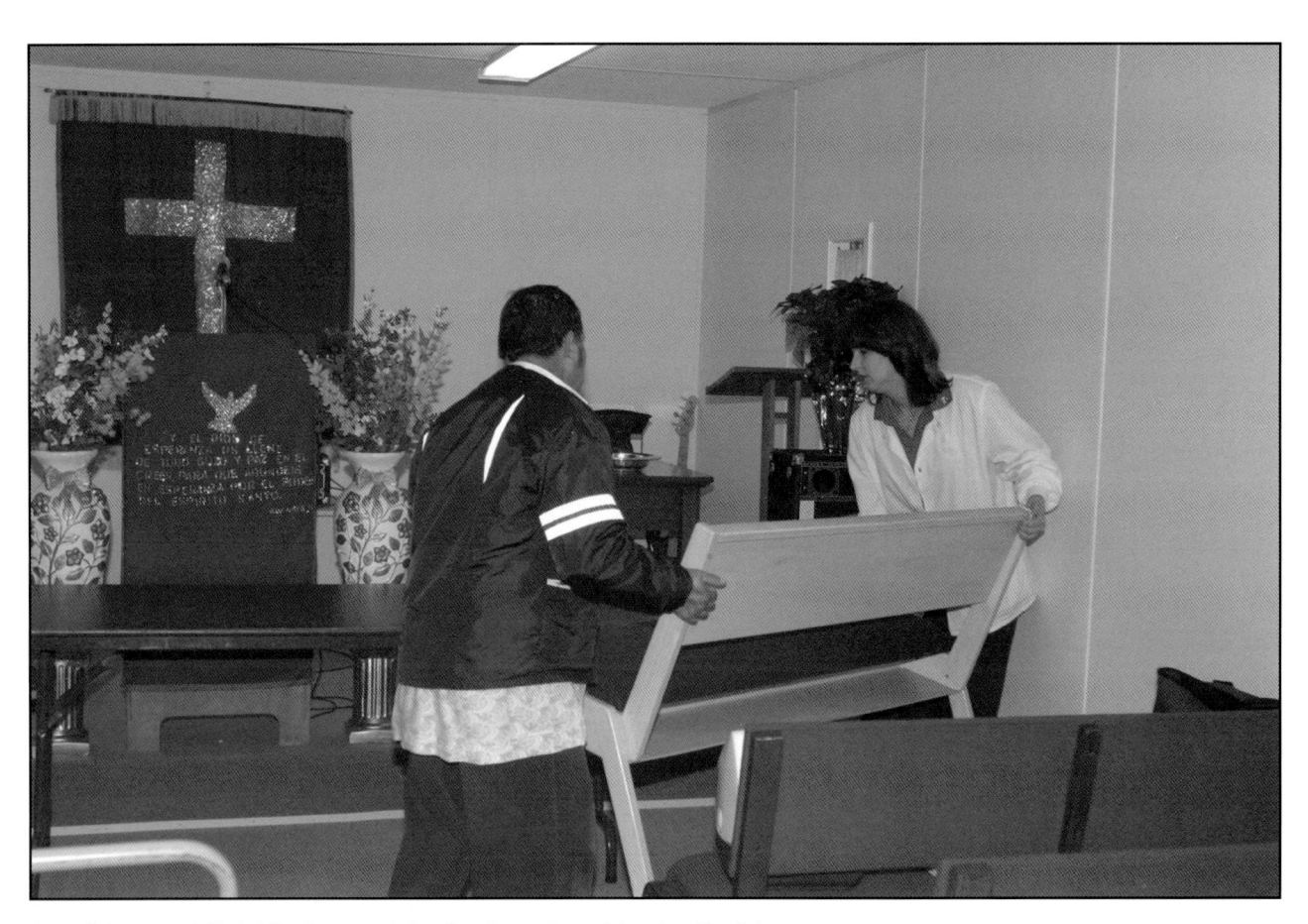

Juan Cabrera and Christi Doyle convert the church sanctuary into a health clinic.

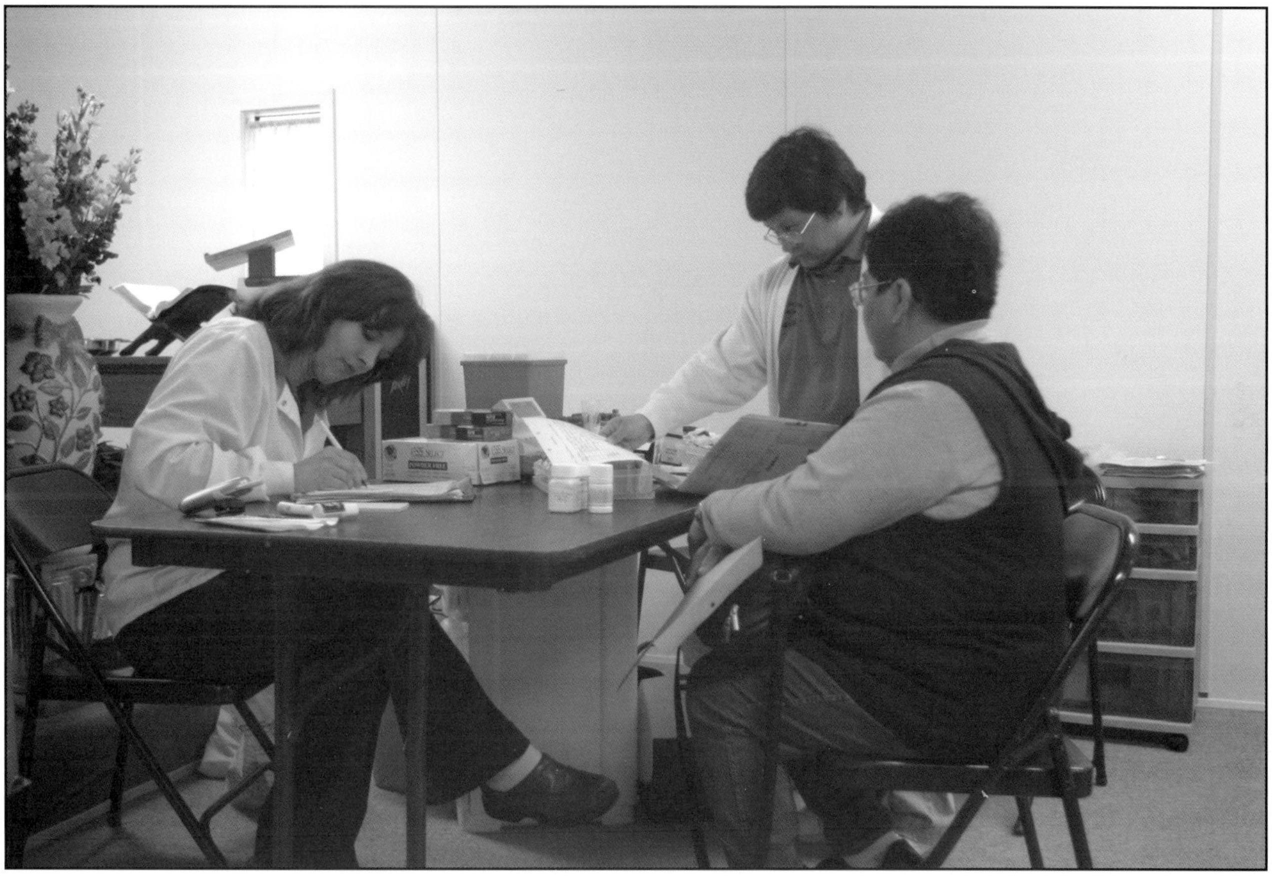

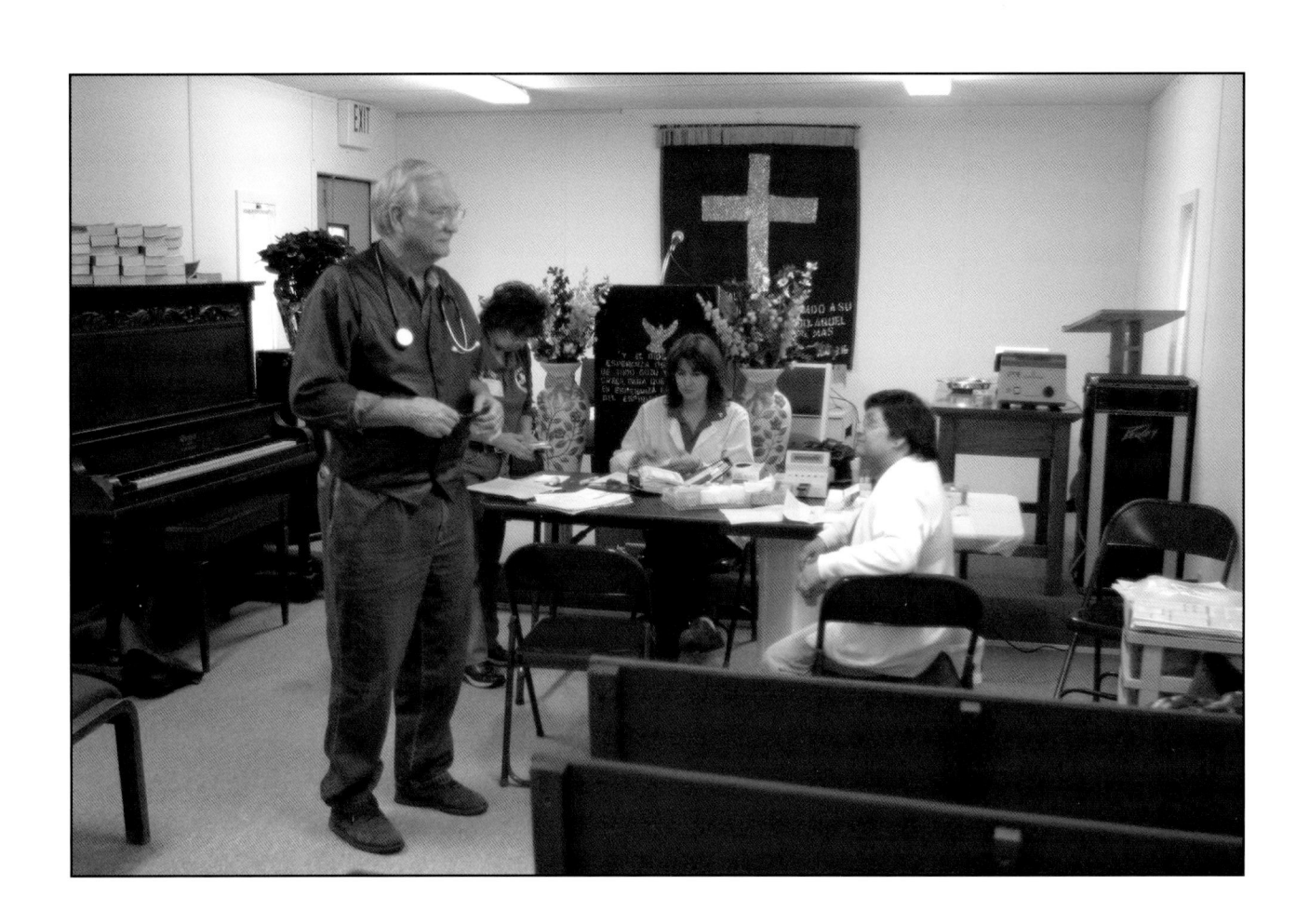

The clinic is open to all residents of Texas, documented or undocumented. Services—examination, some laboratory work, and prescription drugs—are free to those at or below 100 percent of poverty. Others are charged according to a sliding fee scale based on ability to pay. Nearly all patients fall into the former category.

"Most of these people," says Sciarrini, "have essentially nothing."

In addition to their chronic poverty, most of the patients are struggling with chronic diseases. Indeed, because the van stops in each community only once a month, the focus is on chronic rather than acute conditions. It does little good to wait a month to see the doctor for a cold or the flu.

"People come from another culture and try to adapt to our culture and our diet and they don't adapt well," says C. Duane Tisdale, D.O., one of three physicians who go out with the crew on a rotating basis. "We see a lot of degenerative diseases related to lifestyle—things like diabetes and hypertension."

And many of the patients, says Tisdale, who speaks both English and Spanish, return month after month, allowing him to establish a long-term doctor-patient relationship with them.

And that, according to Scott, is yet another highlight of the program. "If people don't have insurance or income to pay for a doctor, the places that are available to them are so institutional and so impersonal," she says. "That's not how this is. They really do have relationships with the people."

Results

The van brings care to some twenty patients at each of its monthly visits to the eight sites. To date, nearly 3,000 patients have been seen. Approximately 300 to 400 each year are new patients. Some, says Sciarrini, had not seen a doctor in twenty-five years.

Impressive as those results are, no one involved in the program sees it as a permanent solution to the needs of the region's underserved population. So, in addition to providing treatment, the program seeks to find permanent medical homes for its patients, referring them to clinics that will see them and helping to enroll them in programs for which they are eligible.

"We see a lot of degenerative diseases related to lifestyle—things like diabetes and hypertension."

C. Duane Tisdale

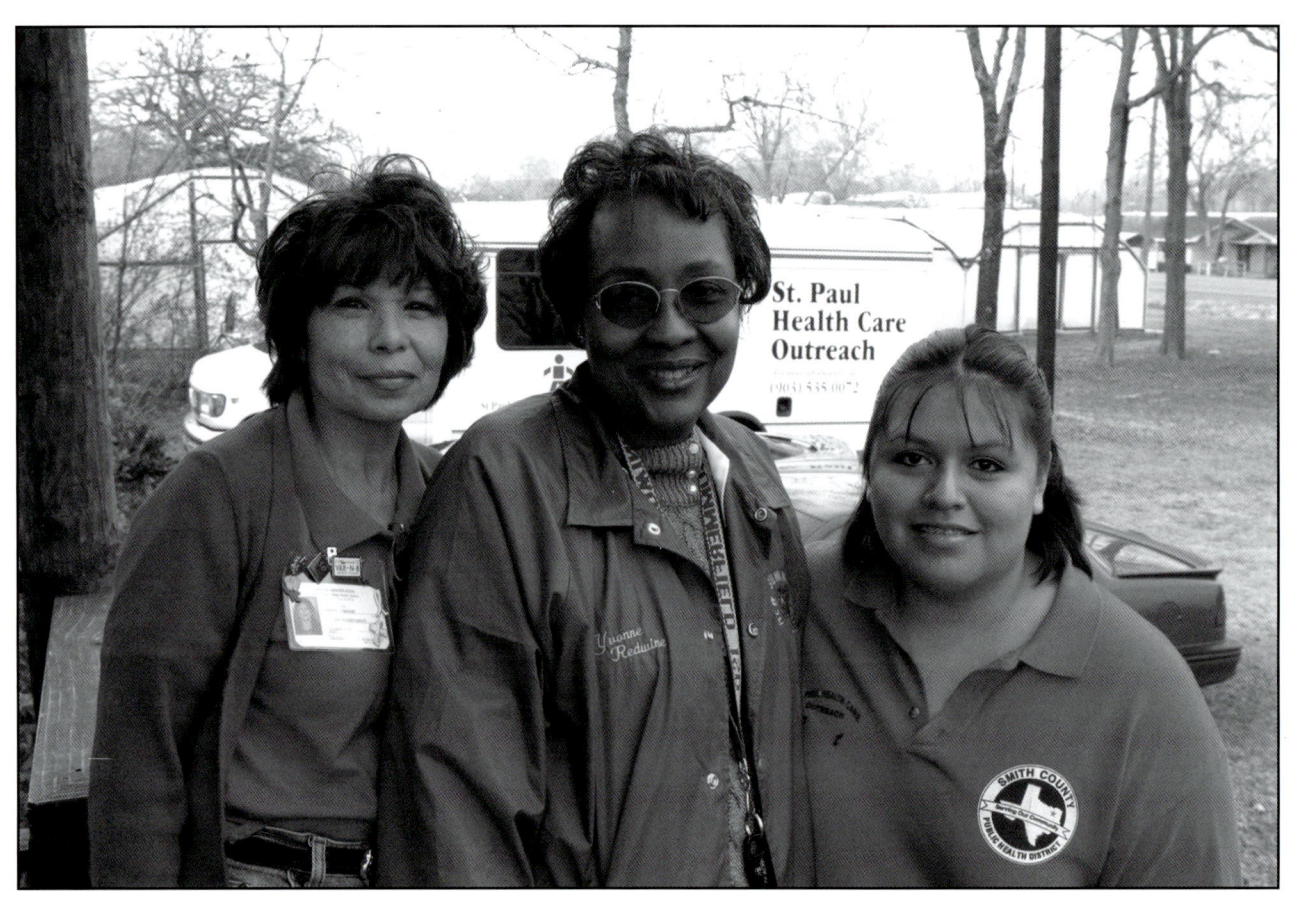

(l to r) Ramona Gonzalez, Yvonne Redwiry, R.N., and Janet Valle have all worked at the mobile clinic.

"We consider it a success if all of our patients leave because we've found them a place to go," says Sciarrini. "Once we've done that, we can move on to another place to start again. And I don't think there's a problem with finding additional sites."

Serving additional sites will, of course, require additional resources. Specifically, it will necessitate a second crew to hit the road while the first crew attends to case management—referrals, laboratory results, etc.—back at headquarters. Sciarrini is searching for the funds.

In the meantime, the van rolls on.

Just the Facts

Purpose

The St. Paul Health Care Outreach Van takes medical care to underserved areas in rural east Texas.

Target Population

The program serves poor, uninsured residents in an eight-county region.

Partners

The van is a collaborative effort of the St. Paul Children's Foundation, the Northeast Texas Public Health District, the state of Texas, and rural community churches, with additional support from city and county government, private foundations, and pharmaceutical companies.

Budget

It cost $82,000 to purchase and equip the van and approximately $235,000 in annual operating costs at this time.

Results

Through the van, some 3,000 patients have been seen to date, most of whom would not otherwise have had care.

For more information, contact Nick Sciarrini, Director, Northeast Texas Public Health District, (903) 535-0036.

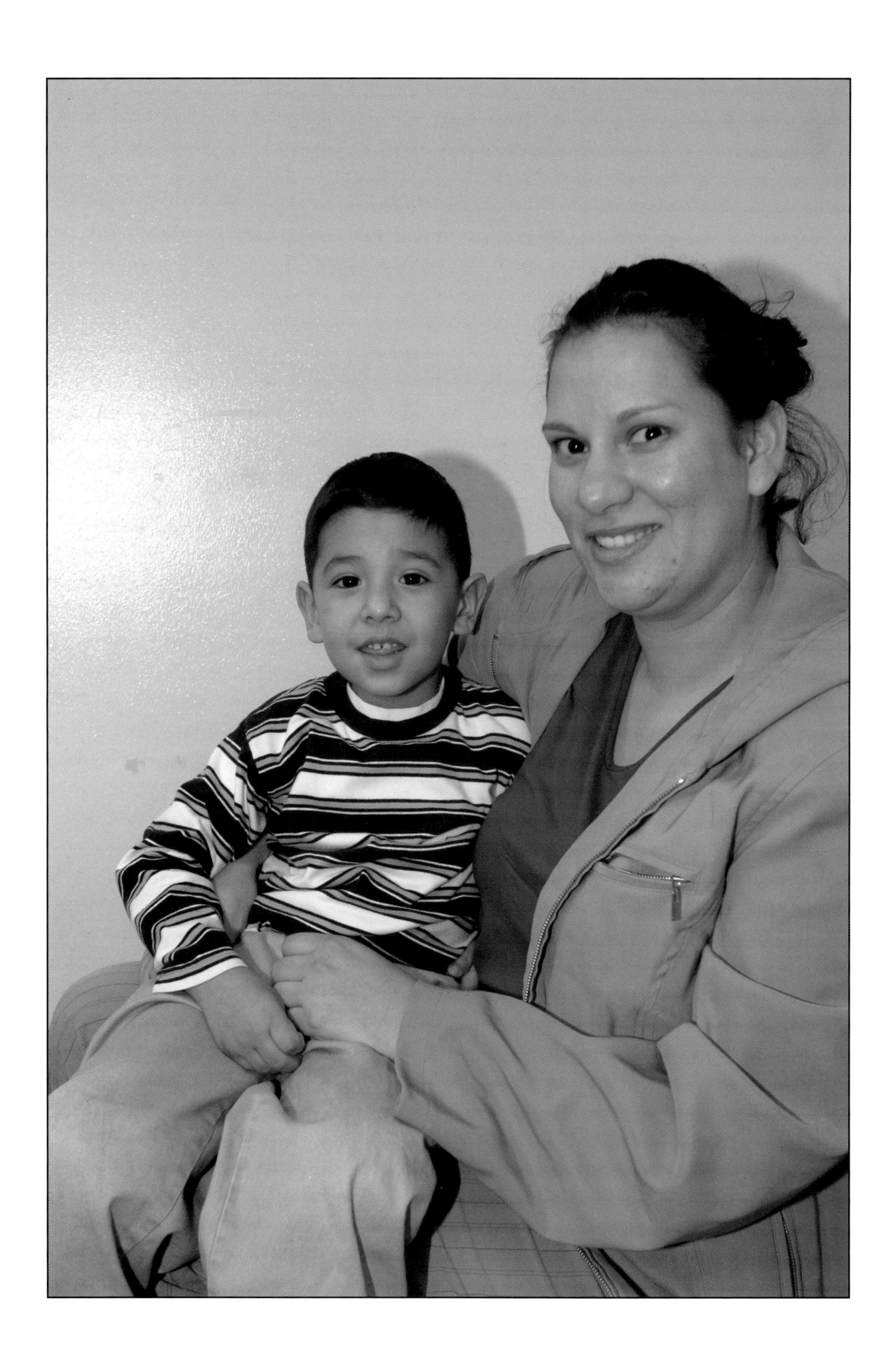

Restoring Smiles:
Central California Dental Surgicenter

Five-year-old Elijah Torres sits quietly on his mother's lap—until he sees the needle. His mother, Eunice Gomez, tightens her grip and does her best to control and console him while the dental anesthesiologist goes for the stick. Once in his bloodstream, the drug works quickly. Elijah's teary eyes get heavy; his flailing body goes limp. Two minutes later, it's time for the dentist.

So it goes, eighteen times a day at the Central California Dental Surgicenter (CCDS) in Atwater, California. Children and developmentally disabled adults, for whom enduring dental treatment is at best difficult, at times impossible, are provided with comprehensive care—from routine examinations and cleaning to complete dental reconstruction—in one sitting, sound asleep, blissfully unaware of the procedures.

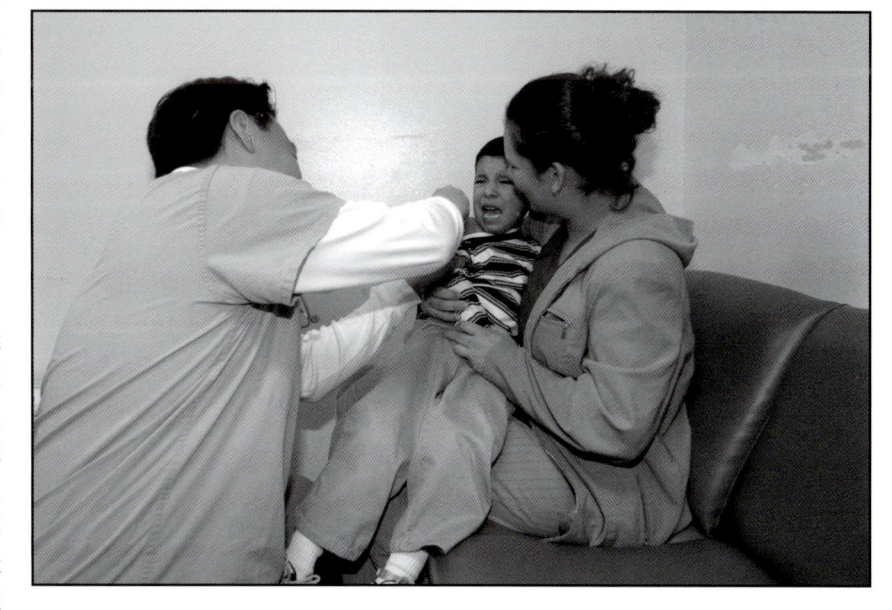

The patients, many of them children of agricultural workers, come from as far as 250 miles away and some of the state's most remote rural places. They come also from some of the state's poorest places.

"Everybody thinks everybody in California is rich. And then you look at the Central Valley…." says L. Ned Miller, CEO of Bloss Memorial Health Care District, one of two partner entities in CCDS. According to Miller, the unemployment rate in Merced County fluctuates between 14 and 16 percent. "This is a very poor area," he says.

Photo opposite page: Elijah Torres and his mother, Eunice Gomez.

53

CCDS Director of Nursing Vickie Kasprzyk, R.N., concurs. "Of the 35,000 children in our area," she says, "47 percent are at or below 200 percent of poverty. We have nothing but poor children here."

The Program

Begun in 1999, CCDS is one of only four programs in the state offering full dental treatment under general anesthesia to children and disabled adults. It is a partnership between Bloss—a not-for-profit public entity that also runs three Rural Health Clinics, an adult day center, and a wound care clinic—and a for-profit private entity owned by Larry Church, D.D.S. How that partnership came about is a story of happy coincidences.

In 1994, the U.S. government closed Atwater's Castle Air Force Base, leaving a $250 million-a-year hole in the local economy. The closure, however, also left the community with real estate, buildings, and equipment that could be used in redevelopment. Included in the inventory was the base hospital, which the U.S. Air Force first leased and then later gave to Bloss Memorial Health District. That gift, says Miller, made a huge difference to the area's health care infrastructure.

"We walked in this empty building, opened up, and doctors and specialists started coming in. It's given access to these low-income farm and factory workers to some specialty care that otherwise would be almost impossible for them to get."

In the meantime, Church was on the faculty at southern California's Loma Linda University, which has its own dental surgicenter. The dentist was growing a bit restless with the slow pace of academic life when a mutual friend of his and Miller's suggested that the two meet. They did, and the partnership was forged: Church brought his knowledge of dentistry in general and dental surgicenters in particular, Miller provided space and a way to access public funds.

To say there was a ready demand for the service would be an understatement. CCDS had a waiting list of 250 children before ever opening its doors.

Why? The surgicenter takes care of patients that no other dentist wants or is equipped to handle, says Church, those who need extensive treatment, those who cannot be treated without anesthesia, those who have a low

> *"Of the 35,000 children in our area, 47 percent are at or below 200 percent of poverty. We have nothing but poor children here."*
>
> Vickie Kasprzyk

income and are covered only by Medicaid or other public insurance (95 percent of CCDS's patients have public insurance), and, occasionally, those who cannot pay at all.

"That's really our mission," he says.

"In this area...the amount of decay is just unbelievable. Kids running around with baby bottle tooth decay...come in and need ten pulpotomies, which is like a baby-tooth root canal, and ten stainless steel crowns. Some need twenty. Every now and then we get a kid that only needs a few fillings, but they're at the age where they can't be treated conventionally. If a kid can be treated conventionally, we refer them to a regular dentist. We only treat patients that require general anesthesia."

A hospital, says Church, could charge as much as $6,000 for such treatment. "We get all these patients that don't have anything and they get it all for free basically."

In spite of that, CCDS makes a profit. It does so by specializing in what it does. That, in turn, allows staff to work faster and more efficiently and thus treat a high volume of patients—eighteen a day (nine per dentist), 300 to 400 a month.

"You can do a lot of work in a short amount of time," says Kasprzyk, "because the kid is unconscious and...not wiggling around."

Revenue is also helped by the fact that some patients have private insurance, which reimburses at a much higher rate than public.

Finally, because CCDS is a public-private partnership, it receives grants to help cover costs.

And unlike most rural practices, CCDS has no trouble recruiting and keeping staff, for two reasons. First, CCDS makes it easy on the dentists, dental anesthesiologists, nurses, and assistants with whom it contracts by keeping them busy and, therefore, paid; taking care of the paperwork hassles; and by giving them a life. No nights, weekends, holidays, or on-call required.

Second, CCDS gives them the opportunity to do truly meaningful work.

The surgicenter takes care of patients that no other dentist wants or is equipped to handle.

Larry Church

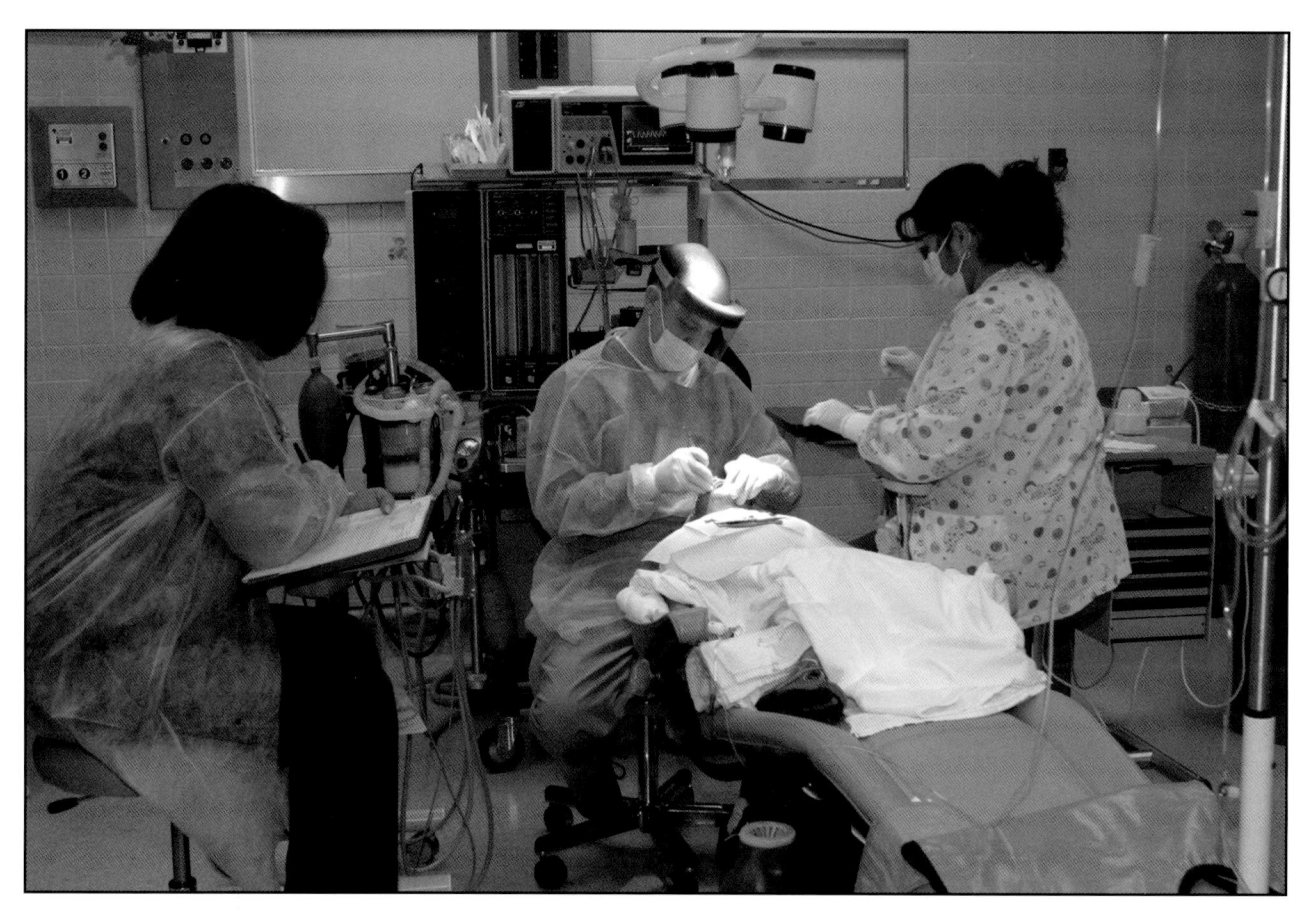

The average time from sedation to the recovery room is about one hour.

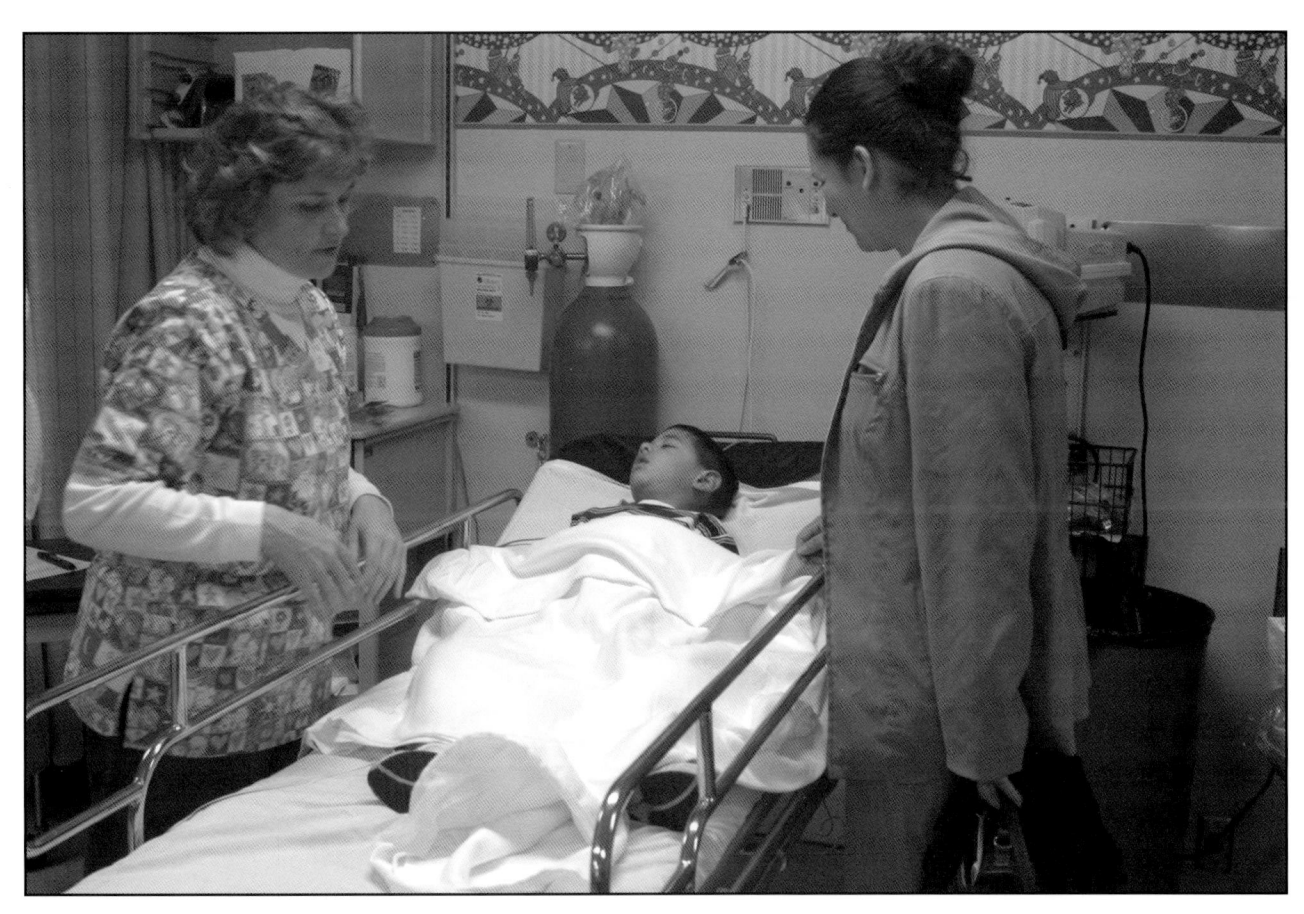

Five-year-old Elijah Torres in the recovery room.

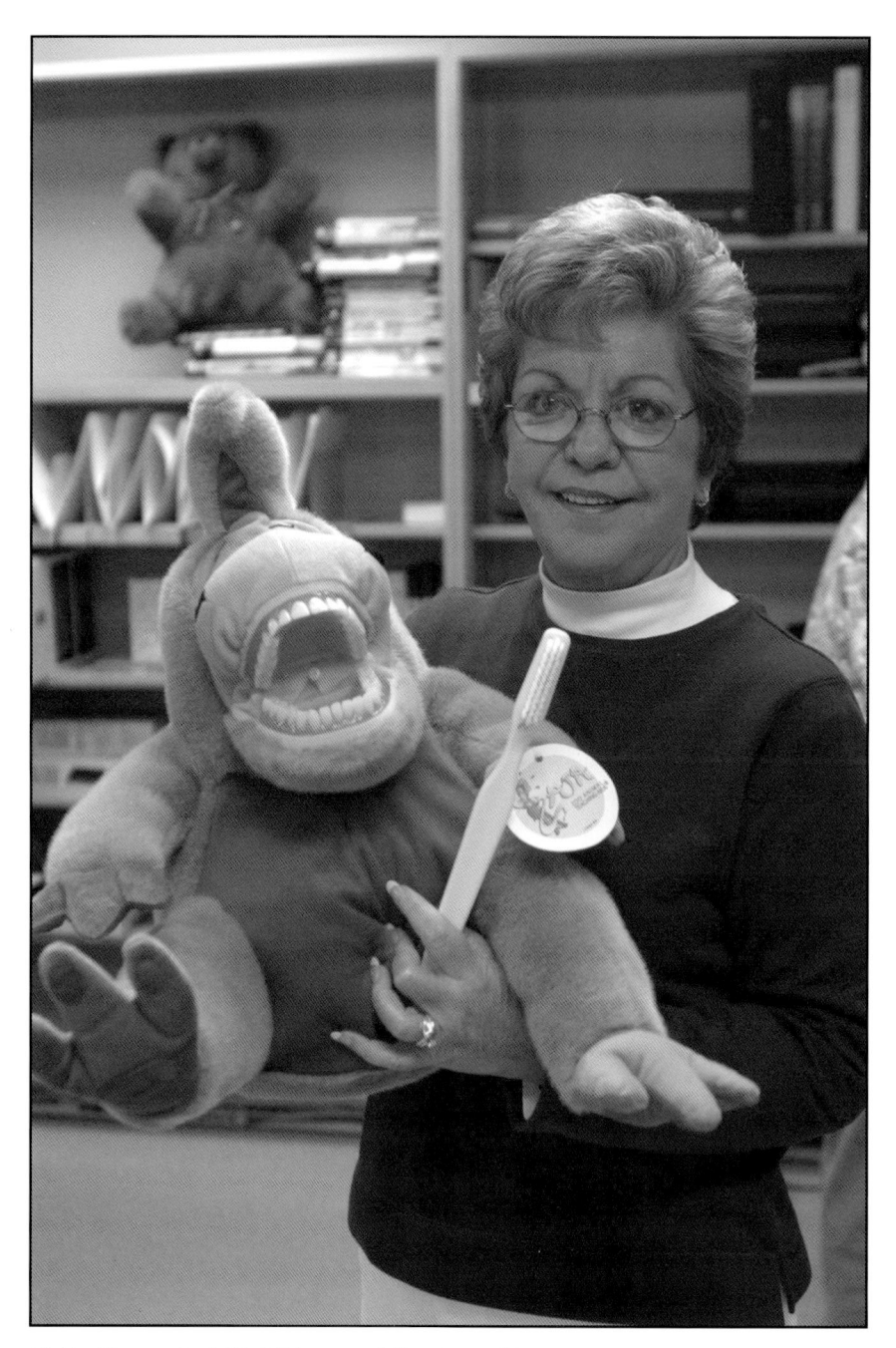

Vickie Kasprzyk, CCDS Director of Nursing, with props used at monthly outreach programs on proper dental care.

"You're helping people that may not get help easily from any other means," says Dennis Clark, D.D.S. "A lot of us do this because of our Christian values. For me, that's important."

Dental assistant Linda Owens expresses similar satisfaction. "We see a lot of things that I don't think a general dentist would see," says Owens. "In a way, a lot of this decay is a form of neglect…and borderline abuse. Some of them are very fragile and we see the signs…. If their mouth is being neglected, then a lot of other things are being neglected. It breaks your heart…."

"At the end of the day," says Owens, "I feel like I've helped a lot of families and a lot of kids that wouldn't be seen if it wasn't for this type of facility."

Results

In a mere five years, CCDS has served more than 10,400 patients. Without the surgicenter, the vast majority of those patients—poor, minority children—would not have gotten care. In recognition of that fact, a grant request to California's Healthy Families Program (subsidized insurance for low-income working people) was not only approved, it was increased sixfold, from $51,000 to $314,000.

"They came down, looked at us and who we served, and said 'This is tremendous. Keep up the good work. We're going to give you six times what you asked for.' I was in shock. I was in tears over the phone," says Kasprzyk.

Even more telling than the financial results are the personal ones. Kasprzyk tells of a little Laotian girl she met at one of the community outreach and dental screening events she holds monthly. The four-year-old's teeth were decayed to the point of endangering her health. Feverish, her gums were infected and full of pus. Her condition was so bad, says Kasprzyk, that "I nearly called Child Protective Services." Instead, she scheduled her for treatment.

The child was living with her grandmother. She was poor, uninsured, and, because of bureaucratic red tape, was falling through the cracks.

"At the end of the day, I feel like I've helped a lot of families and a lot of kids that wouldn't be seen if it wasn't for this type of facility."

Linda Owens

CCDS took her case pro bono and gave her nearly $4,500 of treatment.

Across from the nurses' station hangs the thanks they got: a beautiful, handmade tapestry of a Laotian village with a house in the middle signifying the welcome CCDS staff has to come and stay, any time.

It is but one of countless expressions of gratitude they receive, says Kasprzyk, pointing to a file chockful of cards, letters, and pictures. "It makes your life worth living," she says.

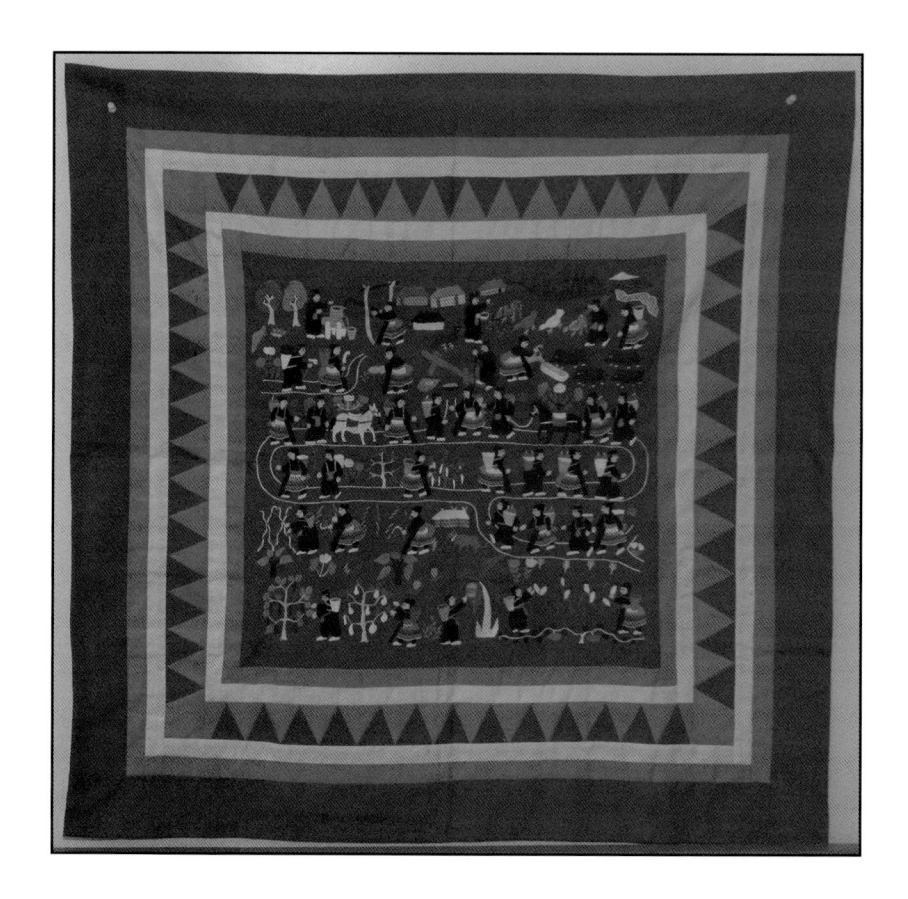

Just the Facts

Purpose

Central California Dental Surgicenter provides comprehensive dental services under general anesthesia.

Target Population

The surgicenter serves patients —children and developmentally disabled adults—who live in California's Central Valley and surrounding region for whom conventional dentistry is not an option.

Partners

CCDS is a general partnership between Bloss Memorial Health Care District and Lawrence R. Church, Inc.

Budget

Proprietary data were not made available.

Results

To date, more than 10,400 patients have been served, most of whom would not have otherwise received treatment.

For more information, contact Vickie Kasprzyk, Director of Nursing, at ccdsvickie@secure.elite.net.

Improving Emergency Care:
Comprehensive Advanced Life Support Program—Minnesota

Practicing medicine in rural Granite Falls, Minnesota, sometimes left Dr. Darrell Carter feeling unprepared. Unlike physicians in larger urban settings, rural doctors like Carter often have little support to draw upon, especially in emergency situations when every minute counts. Indeed, fewer colleagues (let alone specialists) with whom to consult and more limited access to specialized technology are the norm in many small, rural places.

"I'm it," says Carter. "The patient's survival or doing well depends on my skill and those of general nurses working with me."

That fact, says the doctor, "ate at me for awhile."

So he did something about it. Carter, a family physician, teamed up with Dr. Ernie Ruiz, then chief of Emergency Medicine at Hennepin County Medical Center, and created the Comprehensive Advanced Life Support program (CALS).

The program, first offered in 1996, trains medical personnel from around the state to anticipate, recognize, and treat life-threatening emergencies. Billed as "a team approach to rural emergency care," CALS is intended for teams consisting of physicians, mid-level practitioners, nurses, and allied health care professionals. While CALS can benefit health care professionals from any setting, it is geared for rural providers, who practice in more isolated and less-equipped communities and thus, out of necessity, must deal with a broad range of emergencies. As part of its focus on rural providers, the CALS provider course is offered at sites around the state to minimize student travel.

The course includes pre-class home study of the CALS provider manual and the completion of a study guide, a two-day, scenario-based provider course covering cardiac, trauma, pediatric, obstetrical, neonatal, airway management; and medical advanced life support; and a one-day benchmark laboratory covering fifty skills necessary for stabilization of critically ill emergency patients. The tuition costs that are paid by the students for the provider course and the laboratory are reduced by a state of Minnesota grant. With successful completion of all components of the CALS program, participants are provided with a CALS certification, which many rural hospitals now accept as a criterion for staff privileges.

According to Carter, other advanced life support courses have been available for many decades, but good as they are, they do not prepare providers to care for the critically ill or injured in communities lacking the latest in diagnostic equipment or subspecialty providers.

"They just didn't fit rural areas," he says.

The CALS program does fit rural areas, so much so that Carter and his team are now looking at taking the program nationwide.

"CALS proves that we can create a system to train for the unknown medical emergencies," says Carter, "even in the smallest communities."

For more information, contact Darrell L. Carter, M.D., CALS Program Director, at dcarter@kilowatt.net.

Meeting Mental Health Needs:
Sowing the Seeds of Hope—Seven Midwestern States

Though often something of an afterthought, mental health care is in fact a critical component of overall health care. Unfortunately, gaining access to it in rural areas is a decidedly uphill battle. As a result, many rural residents receive little-to-no support with mental and behavioral health issues. For residents in seven midwestern states, however, that is changing.

Since 1999, and growing out of the dire need for mental health services created by crises on the farm, the Sowing the Seeds of Hope (SSoH) project has provided mental health services to underserved farm populations in Iowa, Kansas, Minnesota, Nebraska, North Dakota, South Dakota and Wisconsin. The program was designed and initiated by the Wisconsin Office of Rural Health and Wisconsin Primary Health Care Association with funding from the federal government's Office of Rural Health Policy and Bureau of Primary Health Care. Today, SSoH operates under the umbrella of AgriWellness, Inc., a nonprofit corporation founded in July 2001 and headquartered in Harlan, Iowa. Partners in each state deliver the services and network with one another to enhance the overall effort.

Though the program varies from state to state, it offers several core services in each state:

• Outreach to identify persons in need of services;

• Training and education of behavioral health care providers, community health workers, natural helpers, the faith community, and others who serve the agricultural population;

• Education about agricultural behavioral health issues;

• Information clearinghouses;

• Crisis hotlines;

• Vouchers for counseling services; and

• Retreats and support group activities for farm couples and families.

According to psychologist, farmer, and director of AgriWellness, Mike Rosmann, Ph.D., farmers live under a tremendous amount of stress. That stress, he says, can distract a farmer from the often-dangerous work at hand, resulting in accidents, injuries, and fatalities.

Stress can also lead to suicide. According to Rosmann, the incidence of suicide in the agricultural community is twice as high as the national average. During the foot-and-mouth disease epidemic in Great Britain a few years ago, the suicide rate among farmers temporarily increased to ten times that country's national average.

As evidence of the success of SSoH, Rosmann points out that during the recent drought in Nebraska, suicides among farmers did not go up.

"I'm convinced that these networks really work," he says.

For more information, see www.agriwellness.org or contact Mike Rosmann, Ph.D., Director, at (712) 235-6100, or agriwellness@fmctc.com.

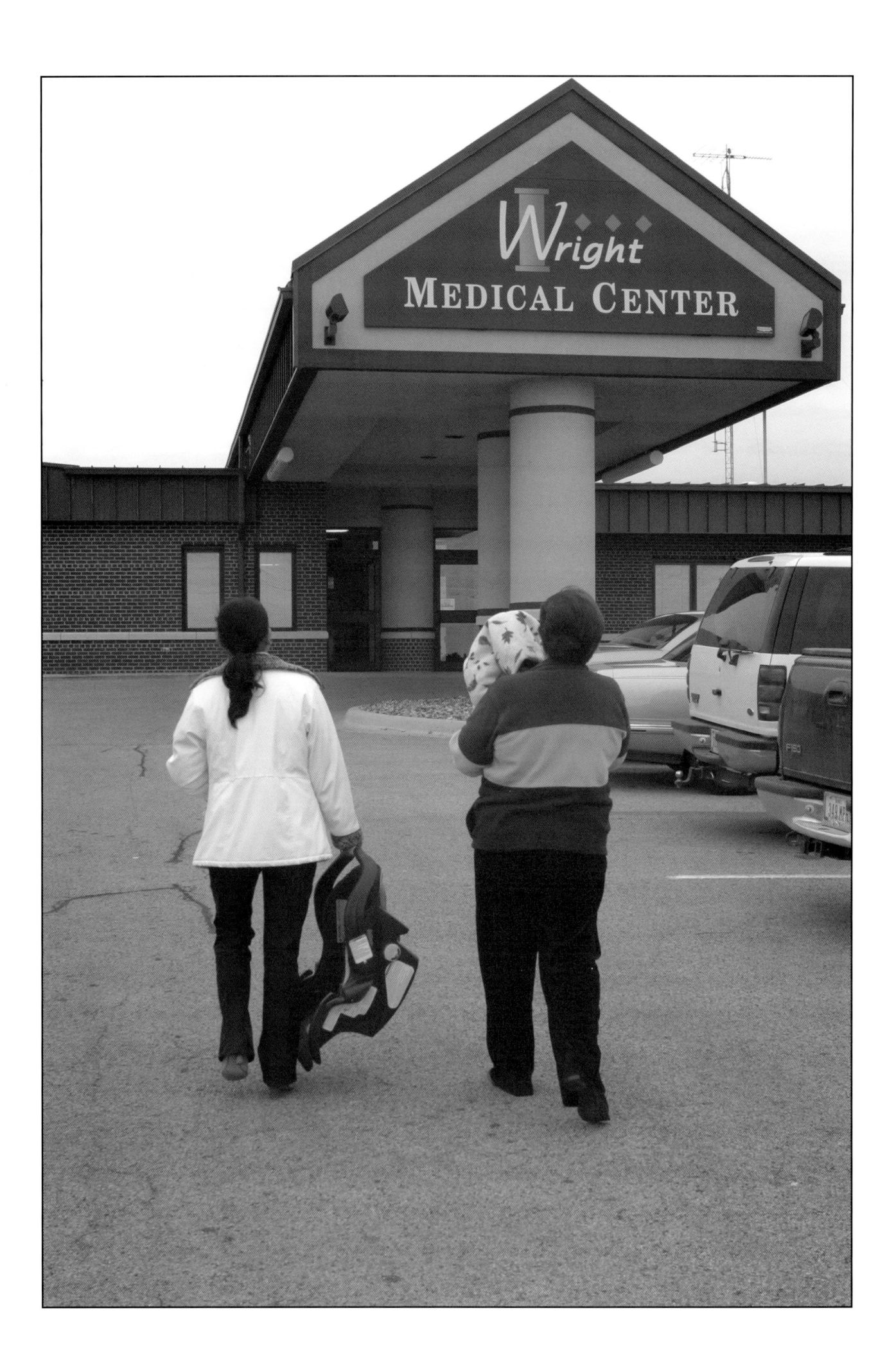

Chapter 3–Meeting Special Needs

The Challenge

Different people have different needs. Some needs go beyond those serviced by traditional health care. Two so-called special needs are on the rise in rural America.

In September 2003, 8.6 million rural Americans had no health insurance. Countless others had less-than-adequate coverage. Without adequate coverage, these people—many, but not all, of them living near or below the poverty level—often forego medical care. When they do seek care, their conditions are generally worse, often urgent, and they typically seek it in the emergency room. That costs more money and more lives.

In 2000, the Hispanic population accounted for only 5.5 percent of the nation's rural population. However, growth in the Hispanic population accounted for 25 percent of all rural population growth from 1990 to 2000. In some counties of the Midwest and Great Plains, the growth in the Hispanic population was the only growth. Many of these people come from Central and South America, speak little or no English, and are poor and uninsured. Some are in this country without documentation. This relatively new demographic phenomenon has caught many rural areas off guard and left them struggling to meet the special needs of new immigrants.

The Innovations

While medical providers have always provided charity care to those who cannot afford to pay, the crush of the rising number of uninsured has left many providers unable to keep up with demand. In Marquette, Michigan, the Medical Care Access Coalition has systematized free care to the poor and uninsured in such a way that patients get the care they need, as well as the dignity they deserve, while physicians, dentists, and other care givers are relieved of many of the burdens of free care and thereby enabled to give more, and more efficiently.

Similarly, Wright Medical Center in Clarion, Iowa, has lent its support to two institutions that care primarily for Hispanic immigrants who came to work in the region's agricultural processing industry. The result of that support is better, more comprehensive care for the immigrants, better financial health for the health care system, and better community for all.

Photo opposite page: Wright Medical Center, Clarion, Iowa.

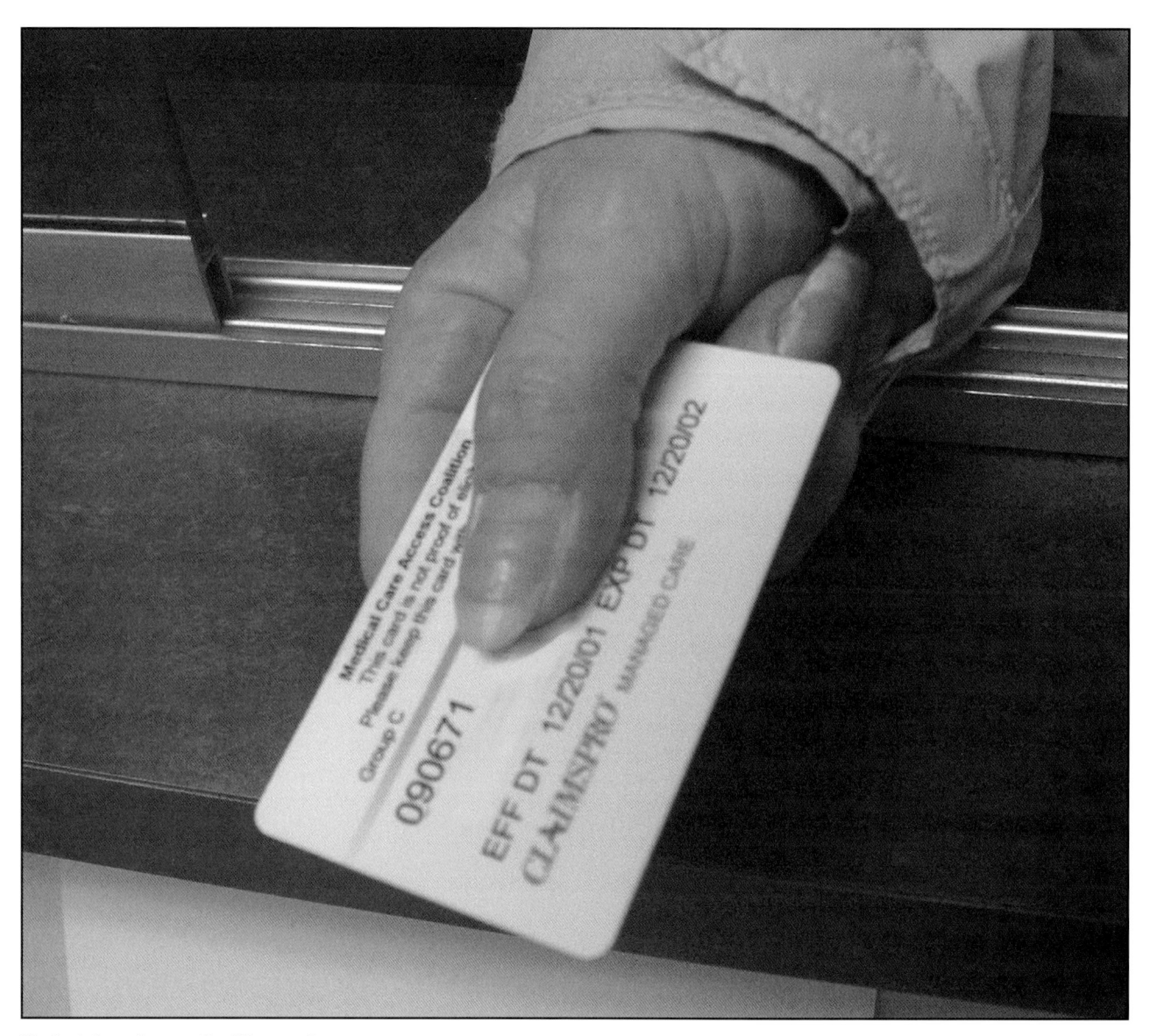

Medical Care Access Coalition card.

Helping the Poor and Uninsured (and Their Doctors): Medical Care Access Coalition—Michigan

When Margaret Couture was laid off in 2001 from a job where she had worked for 16 years, she lost not only her paycheck and a measure of self-esteem, she also lost her health insurance. Insurance or no, however, the pacemaker in her chest has to be checked every other month and her prescription medications have to be taken. The question for Couture: how? How—with no income save her husband's $908 a month Social Security payment and no insurance—could she pay for the medical care she needed? At 58, she doesn't qualify for Medicare; she doesn't qualify for Medicaid; and buying insurance on her own is simply too expensive.

"I felt bad not working and not being able to provide my own insurance. ... I needed something."

Margaret Couture

As a result, says Couture, she reduced her own medications and ignored the pacemaker for a couple of years. "I felt bad not working and not being able to provide my own insurance .... I needed something."

Couture is not alone in needing something, namely access to medical care. Some 7,200 residents (nearly 12 percent of the population) of Marquette County in Michigan's Upper Peninsula are uninsured. On top of that, 3,200 of those uninsured people live at or below 200 percent of the federal poverty level. With little money and no insurance, these people live in constant danger of medical catastrophe and financial ruin. Many seek care only when their conditions warrant a trip to the emergency room. Others may see a doctor (since most physicians provide some charity care), but are unable to pay for prescriptions, laboratory tests, or visits to specialists—things that complete the doctor's care, but things they simply cannot afford.

Neither option is a good one. Fortunately, the Medical Care Access Coalition offers an attractive alternative.

The Program

The Medical Care Access Coalition (MCAC) is a nonprofit organization that enlists and enables health care providers to give free care to Marquette County residents who have no insurance, are between 18 and 65 years old, and have incomes at or below twice the federal poverty rate. MCAC is not an insurance program, but rather a network of providers donating their services. The only cost to eligible participants is a $4 co-pay for prescription medications.

"Health care is not a privilege. It's a right."

Rev. David Mair

MCAC was born in 1999 in a meeting of the Social Education and Action Committee at the First Presbyterian Church in Marquette. Reverend David Mair, interim pastor of the church at the time, stood up and told the group he was angry that the United States has no national health insurance.

"Health care is not a privilege," says Mair. "It's a right. You don't have to earn it. You earn it because you were born."

The room, he says, lit up; and from that spark the idea grew.

While the group was not ready to take on the nation's problems, it was ready to tackle those of Marquette County. It began to study the problems of access to health care and invited people from the community—health care providers, members of other congregations, and anyone else interested—to join in.

Kayla West, a member of the church, a field consultant for the National Health Service Corps, and now vice president of MCAC, knew of a volunteer physician program providing free care to residents in Buncombe County, North Carolina. Members of the group went for a look and liked what they saw. They brought back the idea, adapted it, and launched it. In September 2000, MCAC was incorporated. One year later, it was up and running, serving patients, and growing at breakneck speed.

As Mair puts it, "It floated out of the church and became a community thing."

Indeed, floating out of the church (and the broadly defined faith community) is one of the major reasons for MCAC's success. Two previous efforts to serve the county's uninsured and low-income population had failed largely because of turf issues and mistrust. People feared that the previous efforts' leaders—the hospitals and health department—had hidden agendas and ulterior motives. In contrast, the faith community, from which MCAC sprang, was seen as a neutral and trustworthy party to organize the third attempt.

Another major reason for MCAC's success can be summed up in a word: volunteerism. One hundred percent of the county's primary care physicians, 40 percent of its dentists, and a substantial share of medical specialists have joined up to offer free care. Equally as important, the two local hospitals donate laboratory tests, the radiologists give x-rays; and the pharmacists and pharmaceutical companies help with prescriptions. Together, the services offer a complete continuum of care.

Sue LeGalley, former president of MCAC, and her cardiologist-husband were part of the original committee and helped recruit many of the physicians to participate. "It was just magical how everyone came together to bring their piece of the puzzle," she says. "When asked, no one said 'no'."

The key to getting providers to participate, she says, is that it is entirely voluntary. "You take the spirit away from people when you mandate," says LeGalley. "The doctors, nurses, and dentists feel good about it because no one says you have to do this."

That said, she also points out that providers are already giving free care, and that by joining the coalition, they not only help ensure that the time giving that free care is well spent, they also relieve themselves of the huge administrative burdens and costs that free care entails—sending bills that go unpaid, for example, takes time and money, $7 to $11 per bill sent.

In short, MCAC helps providers help others and help themselves. Specifically, it screens patients to determine who really is in need; fills out time-consuming forms so doctors' offices do not have to; and gets patients the prescription drugs, laboratory tests, x-rays, and specialty care that the doctors prescribe and that complete the necessary continuum of care.

"Our program really does empower the doctors to do what they've always wanted to do," says West. "It allows them to take care of patients the way they want. They know if they prescribe something or order a test, that the

One hundred percent of the county's primary care physicians, 40 percent of its dentists, and a substantial share of medical specialists have joined up to offer free care.

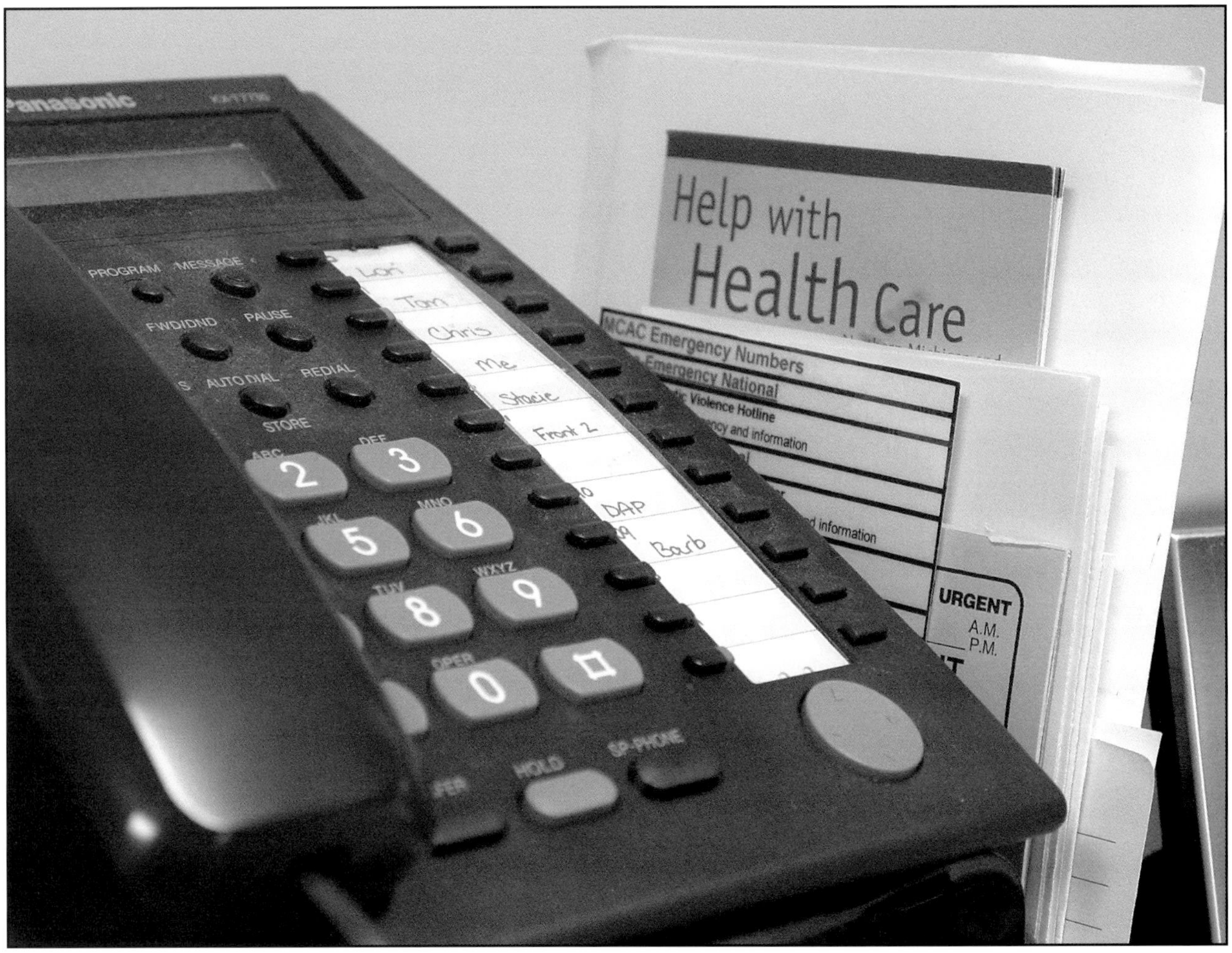
Panasonic
PROGRAM
MESSAGE
FWD/DND
PAUSE
AUTO DIAL
REDIAL
STORE
Lori
Tom
Chris
Me
Stacie
Front 2
DAP
Barb
HOLD
SP-PHONE
Help with Health Care
MCAC Emergency Numbers
Emergency National
URGENT
A.M.
P.M.

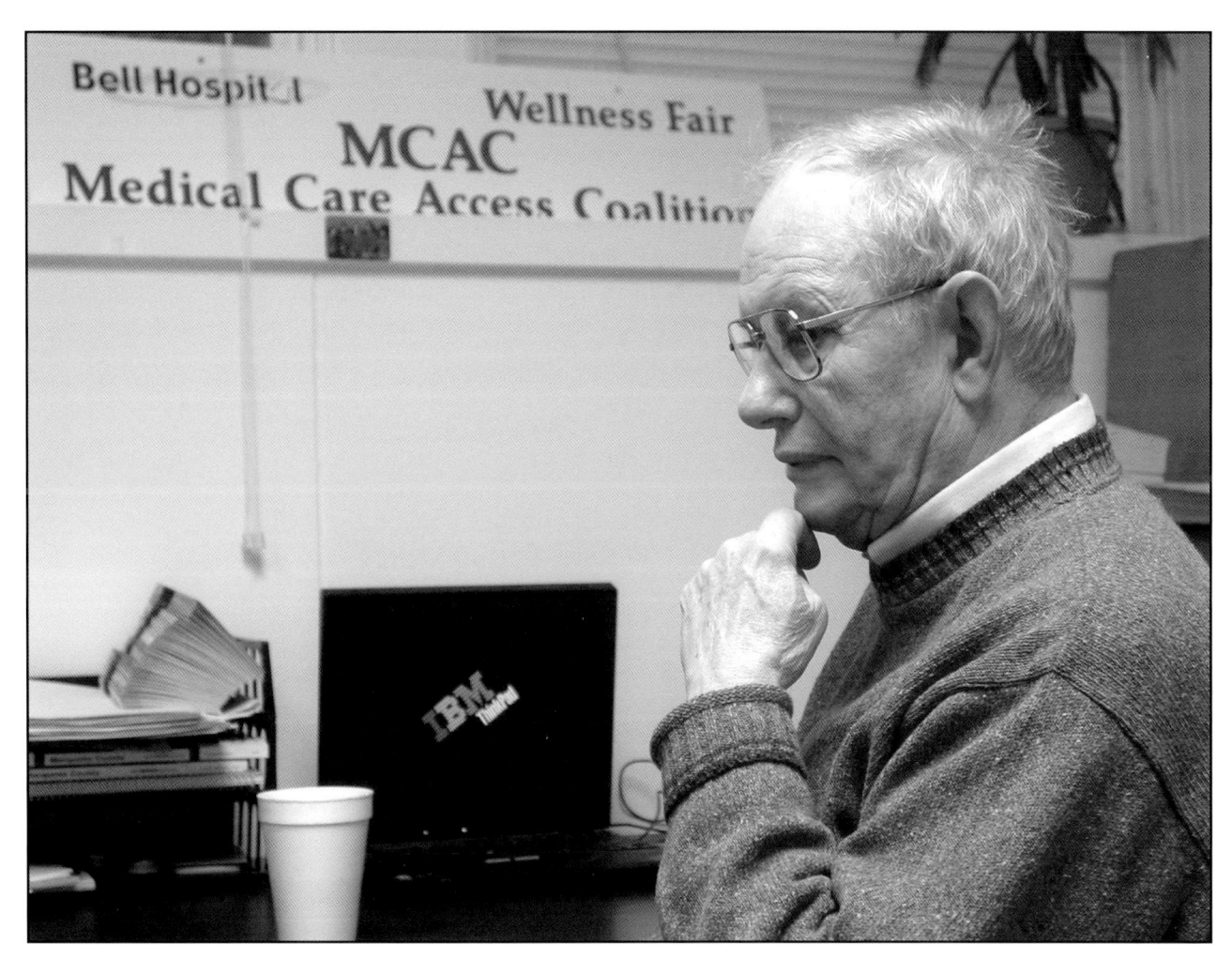

Rev. David T. Mair

Another key to MCAC's success is as simple as a card.

patient will be able to get it. [Doctors] get really frustrated when the people can't get the help they need."

Cary M. Bjork, M.D., is one of those participating physicians as well as an MCAC board member. He sees participation as both the right thing and the smart thing for physicians to do.

"You're probably not doing a whole lot more free care," says Bjork, "but you're avoiding the aggravation of seeing all these uncollectible bills. Nobody likes to send patients to collections or small claims court. And you get to do a good thing besides … provide better care and eventually, I think, save the hospitals a lot of money, too."

"Their willingness to help is really a good thing," says Couture. "You know that they want to be doing it. It's not something they're forced to do."

Another key to MCAC's success is as simple as a card. The card, issued to MCAC clients, gains them access to participating providers just like an insurance card. Clients simply walk up to the reception desk, the laboratory, or the pharmacy counter, hand over the card, and receive treatment, just like any other patient, preserving both the patients' privacy and dignity.

The overwhelming response of providers in joining the coalition notwithstanding, office visit slots are not always available. So, MCAC began a weekly clinic to help meet the additional demand and make it easier for patients who work during office hours to come in and see a doctor. The clinic rotates between two sites, broadening geographic access as well.

MCAC President, Karlyn Rapport, cites the clinic as just one example of MCAC's flexibility, perseverance, and willingness to respond to new needs and new opportunities—the final key to its success.

"This has not been a project for the faint of heart," says Rapport. "We have had to take on additional challenges when the opportunity arose and press on regardless. That's an important lesson."

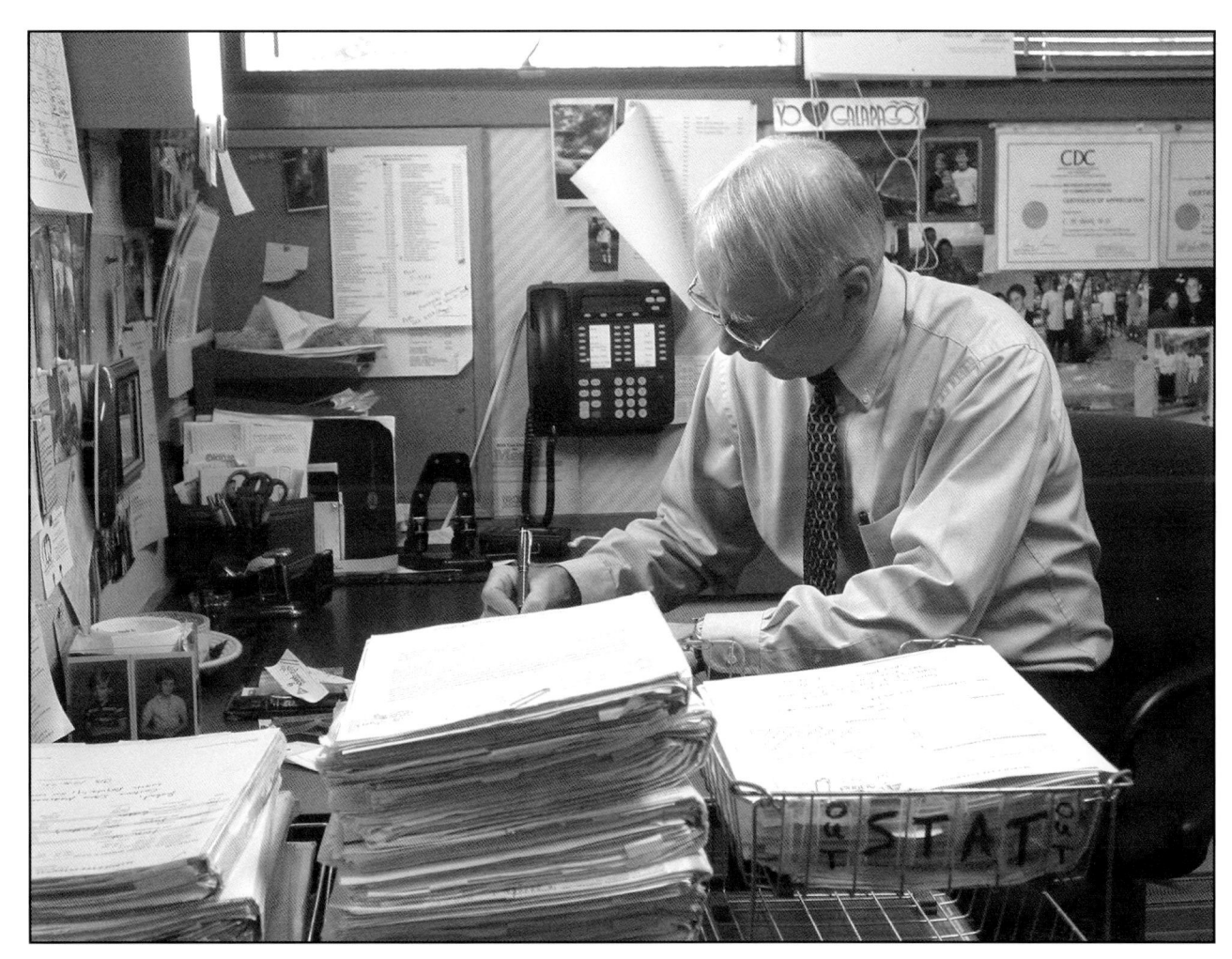

Cary M. Bjork, M.D.

> *"It's been a roller coaster, an amazing ride. You know something is great when it gets blessed everywhere it turns."*
>
> Sue LeGalley

Results

In its short time of operation, MCAC has helped more than 1,400 of the county's 3,200 eligible people. It has done that by enlisting 159 providers and obtaining more than $400,000 of physician services, $46,000 of dental services, and $360,000 prescription drugs.

Not only does MCAC serve those in need, it helps those who are eligible to enroll in programs that provide even more benefits. Some 20 percent of people that apply for MCAC find out that they are, in fact, eligible for Medicaid or the state's Adult Benefit Waivers Program, which the state of Michigan now contracts with MCAC to administer in the Upper Peninsula. In those cases, everyone benefits even more: the person gets even more comprehensive care, providers get paid for providing that care, and the coalition conserves scarce resources.

"It's been a roller coaster, an amazing ride," says LeGalley. "You know something is great when it gets blessed everywhere it turns."

MCAC Executive Director, Tom Viviano, concurs. "It's been almost head spinning," he says of the program's remarkable growth. "We've got a tiger by the tail."

Margaret Couture describes the success of MCAC in much more personal terms. "It made me feel like I was a worthwhile human being," she says. "I don't feel like I've been discarded."

Just the Facts

Purpose

MCAC is a network of health care providers that provide free care to underserved individuals.

Target Population

The program serves Marquette County residents who have no health insurance and have incomes at or below 200 percent of the federal poverty level.

Partners

The Medical Care Access Coalition is a 501(c)(3) organization. The list of its partners is a long one, including churches, synagogues, hospitals, civic groups, the county health department, and state and federal agencies. Initial funding came from the Community Access Program of the Health Resources and Services Administration, U.S. Department of Health and Human Services, and Presbyterian Women U.S.A.

Budget

Annual budget is approximately $275,000.

Results

To date, more than 1,400 people have been served.

For more information, contact Chris Palombo, Director of Outreach and Marketing, cpalombo@penmed.com.

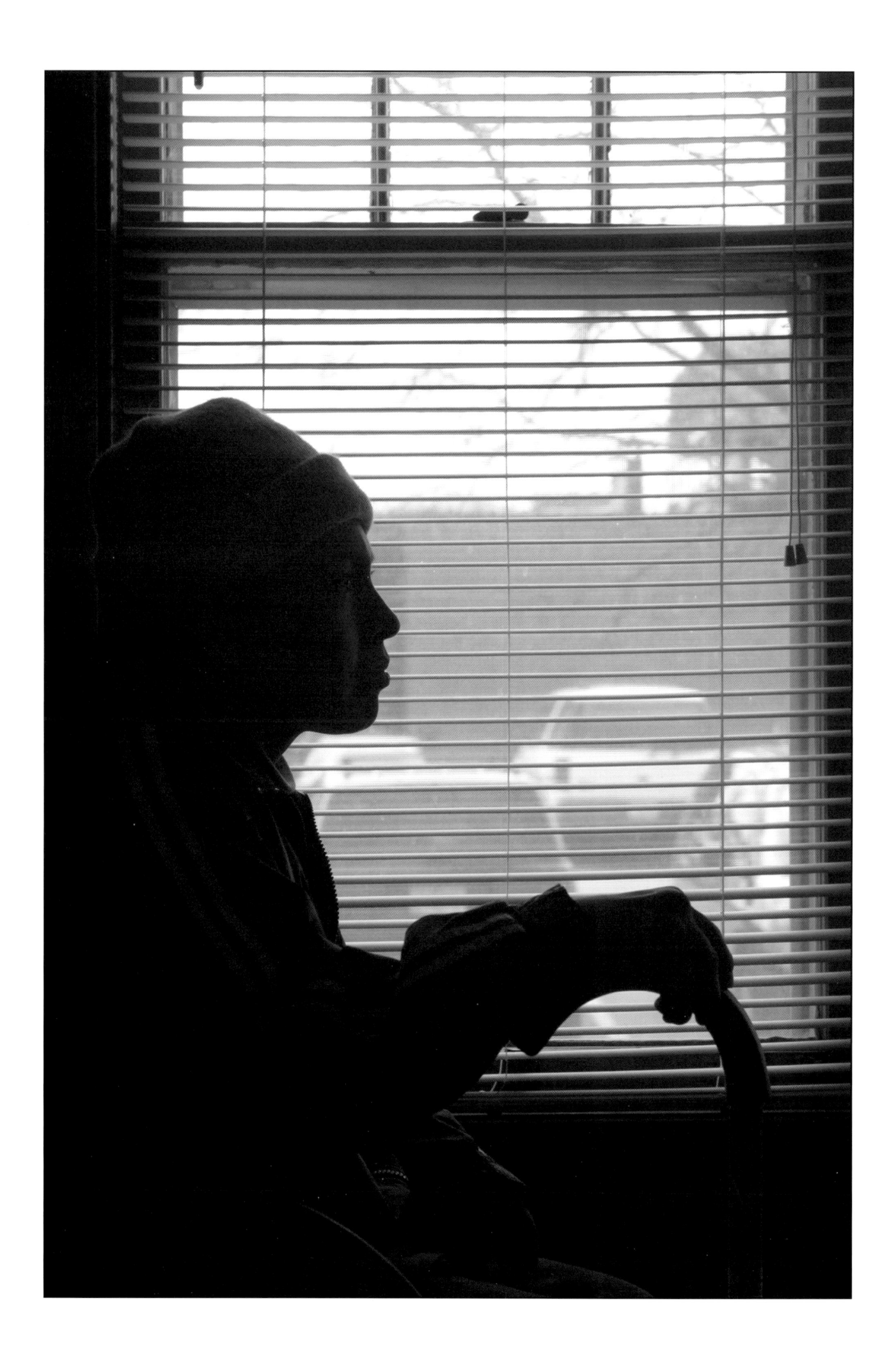

Caring for and about Hispanic Immigrants: Wright Medical Center—Iowa

For Paula, Tomasa, and Geopatica, tiny Clarion, Iowa, is a long way from Mexico, a long way from home. But for these sisters, it is, in many ways, better than home. They, like so many other Central and South Americans who now live in and around this tiny plains community, came north in search of jobs and a better life. The jobs they found at the huge confined animal operations dotting the Iowa landscape. The better life they found in steady work, higher pay, good schools for their children, and last but certainly not least, care at Wright Medical Center.

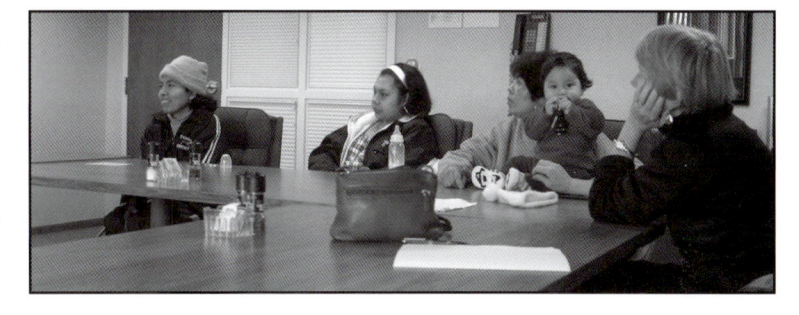

The Program

Wright Medical Center (WMC), a community-owned hospital on the edge of town where lawns turn into cornfields, has welcomed the region's new immigrants, out of a sense of need, but also out of palpable spirit of generosity.

"It's the right thing to do," says CEO Steve Simonin of his hospital's charitable efforts. "The town of Clarion has really embraced the Hispanic community and they've embraced us."

The embrace by WMC takes two forms: the Domestic/Sexual Assault Outreach Center (D/SAOC), which operates out of space donated by WMC, and the Clarion Free Clinic, owned by the hospital, located in it, and run entirely by volunteers, including hospital personnel. Both meet critical needs in the Hispanic community.

Domestic/Sexual Assault Outreach Center. While WMC has been taking care of people for some 50 years, helping provide counseling and other

Photo opposite page: Tomasa Barcenas.

77

"We do whatever we can to help the victims get safe and enable them to become independent and capable of supporting their families. The work we do is not optional."

Joyce DeHaan

nonmedical services to victims of abuse is a recent development. The Clarion center, one of six outreach centers around the state run by a nonprofit organization in Ft. Dodge, opened inside the hospital in 1999. In 2001, the hospital bought a house next door, renovated it, and gave D/SAOC free use of it. The hospital also pays for its utilities and upkeep and helps the center raise funds to operate.

At D/SAOC, victims of domestic and sexual abuse find the help they need to survive: counseling services, support groups, English classes, food, clothing, child care, child advocacy, transportation, and more, all free of charge.

"We do whatever we can to help the victims get safe and enable them to become independent and capable of supporting their families," says Joyce DeHaan, Executive Director of D/SAOC. "The work we do is not optional."

Nor is it easy. Most, but not all, of the victims are Hispanic women who face additional obstacles when it comes to seeking and receiving assistance: language, lack of transportation, and uncertainty over who they can and cannot trust to name a few.

Paula, 41, and Geopatica, 25, are two of those victims. Both work at a nearby egg-packing facility. The work, they say, isn't bad—though they work from 6:30 in the morning until 8:00 at night with no dinner break, no overtime pay, and no benefits. The treatment, they say, is.

Through an interpreter, the women, eyes down and in hushed tones, tell of both verbal and physical abuse at the hands of supervisors: screaming, threats of being fired, and worse.

"They treat us like slaves," says Geopatica, before breaking down in tears. Her older sister quietly nods.

While not a victim of abuse, their sister Tomasa suffers in other ways. Unable to work because of the rheumatoid arthritis that plagues her, the thirty-eight-year-old woman battles the loneliness and isolation of her condition as well as the physical pain and obstacles it presents. She, too, finds help at D/SAOC.

"It takes a lot for them to trust us," says DeHaan. "It takes a while for them to warm up to us. They've been taken advantage of. They fear being turned in as undocumented."

But, she says, it is working. Trust is building. Women are being helped. Paula, Geopatica, and Tomasa are living proof. Further proof comes from an anonymous written testimony that DeHaan shares.

At the Domestic/Sexual Assault Outreach Center, I could finally feel safe. I felt like I was in heaven. Everybody was kind and loving and caring. I felt like I was going to be okay. Through education, support groups, and counseling, I was able to put my life in perspective and my priorities together. I have gotten a job where I can be self-sufficient. I am running a house by myself and raising five really great kids. I always doubted off and on over the past few years if I made the right choice to leave [my husband] until I got the news that my husband's brother stabbed and murdered his wife in front of their two small children. I don't doubt it anymore....Thank you for helping me to save my life.

Clarion Free Clinic. While perhaps less dramatic, the need for care is no less urgent at the Clarion Free Clinic. Wright Medical Center's involvement goes back to the clinic's inception. And credit for its inception, everyone agrees, belongs to one man, Robert McCool, M.D.

McCool was one of four doctors who started the hospital in the 1950s. In the 1990s, spurred on by the increasing number of Hispanic workers in the area in need of free care, and by his and wife Kitty's experiences as medical missionaries on Indian reservations and in other countries, McCool began pushing for a free clinic in Clarion. His work bore fruit in 1995, ten years after retiring from practice, when the doors to Clarion Free Clinic opened. McCool died in 2001, but his partners and WMC have kept his vision and his work alive.

The clinic, open every Tuesday evening, sees some twenty patients a night. Patients—again, most of them Hispanic immigrants—come from as far as fifty miles away. The clinic opens at six o'clock, but patients arrive as much as two hours before.

Julia Hudson, a nurse and translator at WMC, who volunteers at the clinic, says it sometimes "gets pretty hectic." She also says that despite that fact the patients are treated with the utmost dignity. "It's just like if they walked

"At the Domestic/Sexual Assault Outreach Center, I could finally feel safe. I felt like I was in heaven. Everybody was kind and loving and caring. I felt like I was going to be okay."

Anonymous testimony

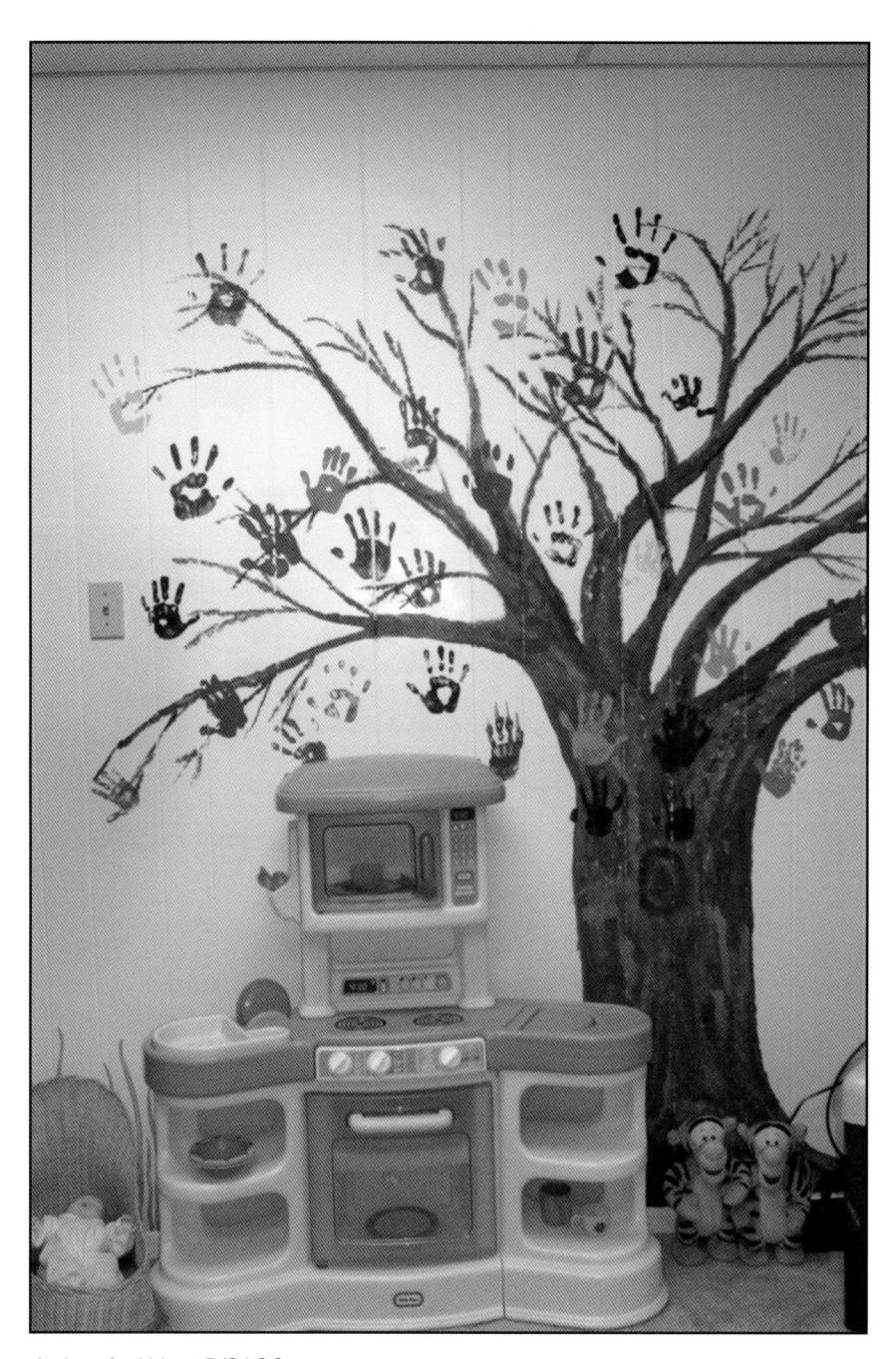

A place for kids at D/SAOC.

in a regular clinic. They sign in. The treatment, everything, is excellent."

The treatment is free of charge and available to anyone without health insurance, whether they are documented or undocumented. (According to staff, "That's none of our business.") Prescription drug samples are given out when available. Discounts are offered at the pharmacy downtown. X-rays and laboratory tests are provided at cost, but sometimes available free of charge for people who cannot afford even that.

Volunteers staff the clinic: one doctor (three share responsibilities on a rotating basis), two nurses, one secretary, and one translator. Most worked closely over the years with McCool and several are now retired, yet continue on.

Phyllis Stupka, R.N., is at the clinic nearly every week. "I've been a nurse since I was 18 years old," says Stupka. "I have done nothing all my life but be a nurse. I'd miss it. I've always said I'm going to quit when I turn 80, but I'm not going to tell anybody when I get there."

Fran Hoyt, who just retired from managing a credit bureau for 30 years, handles the clinic's secretarial duties. She has her own reasons for showing up each week: "I've been in that real poor, poor situation. We've got to help these people."

And help them, they have.

Results

The results of WMC's involvement in the two efforts are evident in the lives of those they have helped, many of whom have nowhere else to turn. Together, the two programs serve more than 1,000 people a year.

The results are also evident in WMC's bottom line.

As Simonin points out, "If we don't see them in the free clinic and if we don't get to them quickly, we're going to see them in the ER, and it's probably going to be a lot more expensive. If we don't have D/SAOC, we're going to see them [in the hospital] as an abuse victim. It's a very proactive way of stemming the violence and decreasing the long-term health costs."

"If we don't see them in the free clinic and if we don't get to them quickly, we're going to see them in the ER, and it's probably going to be a lot more expensive."

Steve Simonin

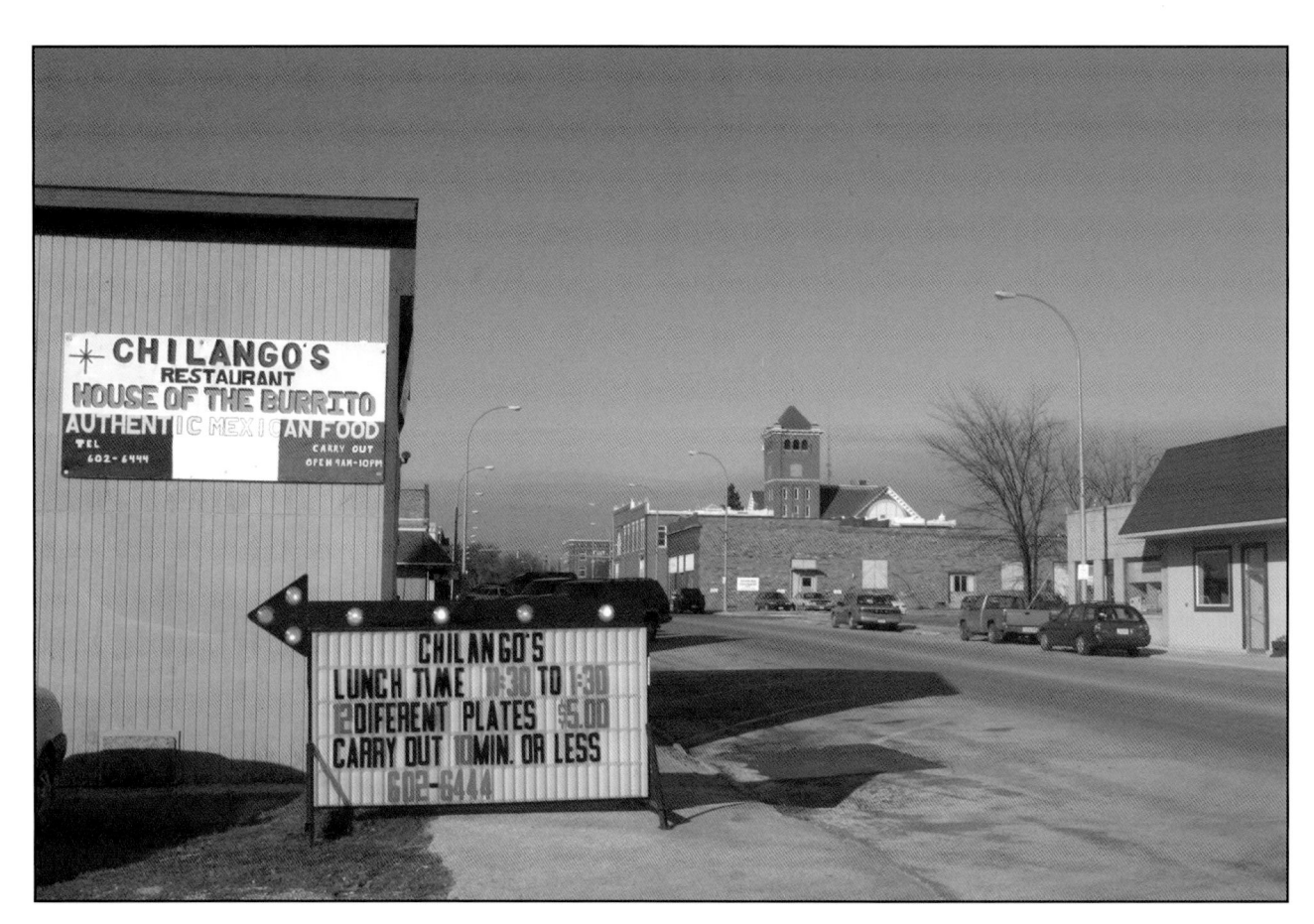

Clarion, Iowa

"In a community like this, we have to take care of these people," he adds. "So if it's not going to come through some of the charitable ways of doing things, it will come through the bad debt and it will tax our services one way or another. It truly is an expansion of our services."

The bottom line is not, however, the bottom line. "We've got to take care of the people," says Simonin. "It's not like we're in this to make money."

According to translator Julia Hudson, that sense of charity pervades the hospital and the community, a community that nine years ago raised $2.3 million in private donations to renovate the hospital. "I have never seen a town or a hospital that is as caring. This hospital goes all out to help. One way or another they bend over backwards to help the patient, the employee, whoever comes in the door. Nobody is looked down upon."

Esperanza Rodriguez Aguilar echoes that sentiment. The 52-year-old grandmother from Mexico came north with her son and his wife in search of work. She comes to the clinic because, with no insurance, she has no place else to go. The closest alternative is in Iowa City, three hours away.

"The clinic has treated me well," she says. "I feel calm, satisfied…because I know they are going to take good care of me. The people are very nice. They try to help us."

"We have got a lot of help here," concurs Paula, "different kinds of help."

Even Geopatica manages a smile.

"I have never seen a town or a hospital that is as caring. This hospital goes all out to help. Nobody is looked down upon."

Julia Hudson

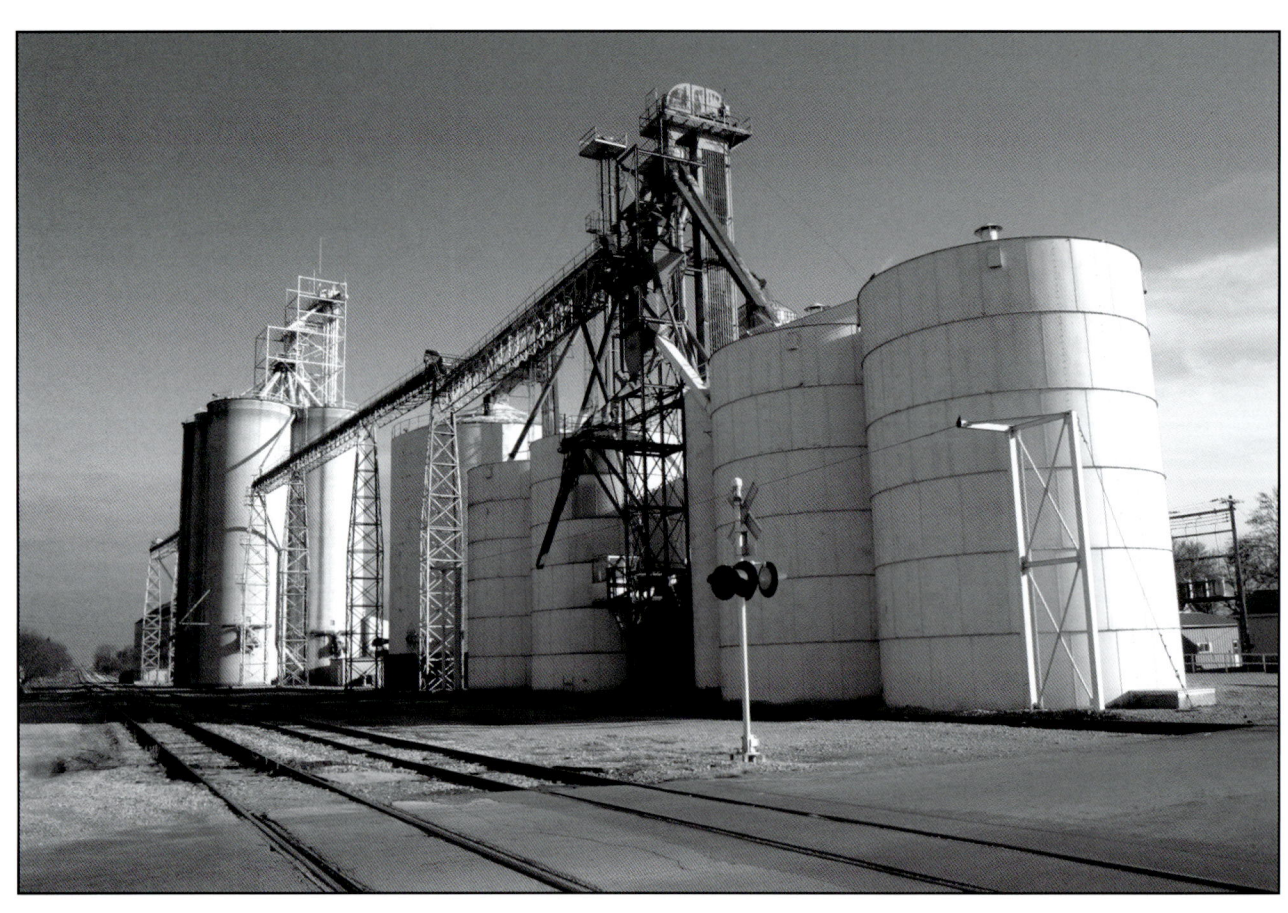

Clarion, Iowa

Just the Facts

Purpose

The Domestic/Sexual Assault Outreach Center provides a range of free services to victims of abuse. The Clarion Free Clinic provides free medical care to uninsured people. Both services are housed at Wright Medical Center.

Target Population

The center and clinic serve all eligible people, but primarily help low-income Hispanic immigrants in the region.

Partners

The outreach center is owned and operated by Domestic//Sexual Assault Outreach Center in Fort Dodge, Iowa. Community partners contributing to both D/SAOC and the free clinic include Wright County, Clarion Community Chest, local churches, and private citizens.

Budget

The annual budget for D/SAOC in Clarion is approximately $120,000 per year. Budget numbers for the free clinic are unavailable since it is staffed by volunteers and laboratory tests are performed on a cost basis.

Results

The D/SAOC served 254 people last year. The free clinic serves approximately 800 patients per year.

For more information, contact Gina Radechel, Marketing and Public Relations Director, at gradechel@wrightmed.com.

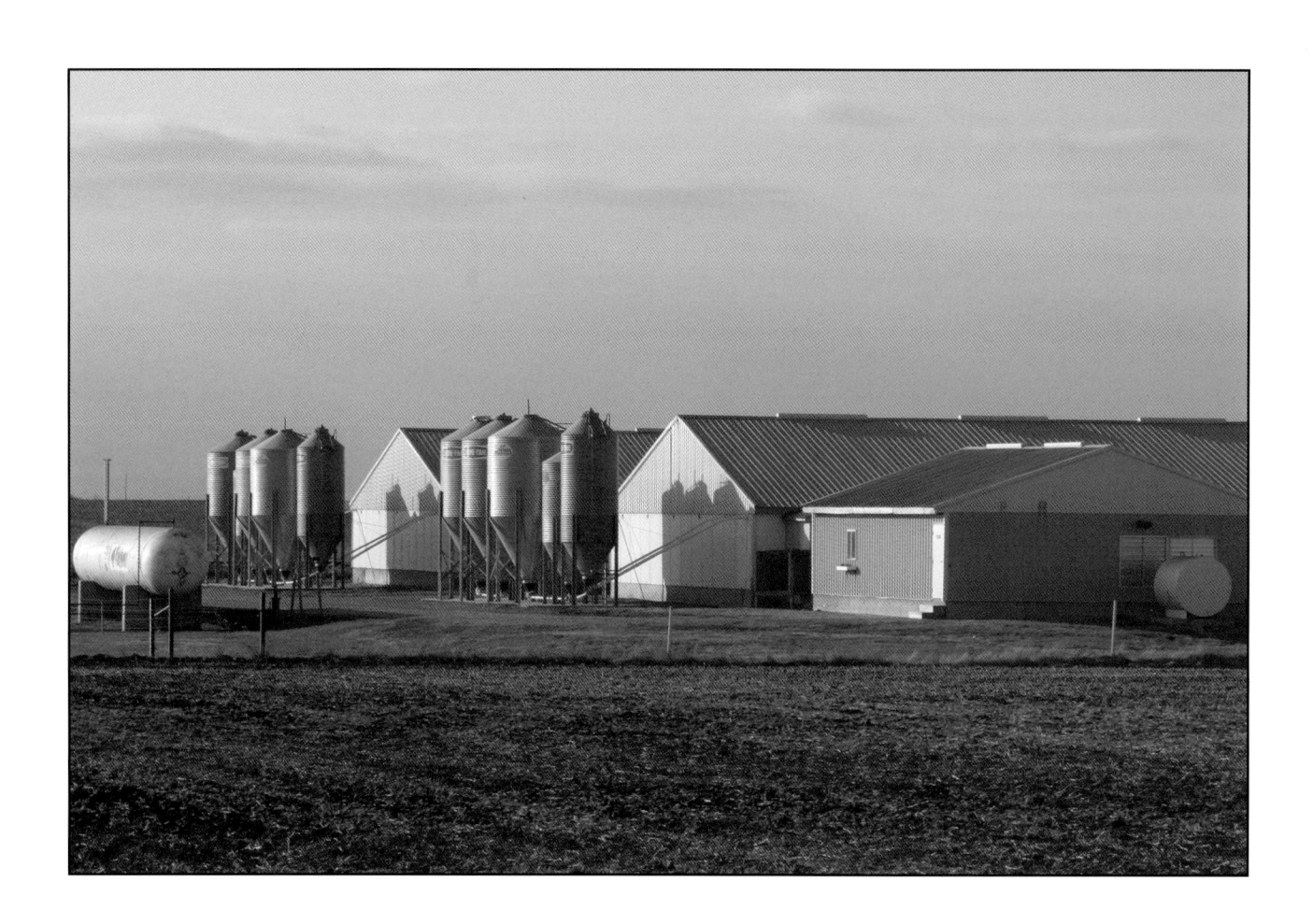

Fighting Diabetes in Kids:
Ho-Chunk Nation Youth Fitness Program—Wisconsin

Type II diabetes runs high among members of the Ho-Chunk Nation in rural Wisconsin. And the youth of the tribe are no exception. Indeed, among the tribe's 6- to 18-year-old population, obesity, which is a major risk factor for the disease, occurs at five times the national rate.

The Ho-Chunk Nation Youth Fitness Program in Baraboo, Black River Falls, and Wisconsin Dells, Wisconsin, however, aims to reduce those numbers and the risk of diabetes. To do that, the project provides at-risk youth with nutrition counseling and exercise training.

On the nutritional front, a pediatric nutritionist performs in-home family assessments, offers opportunities to participate in a community garden, and teaches meal-planning skills. Low-fat cooking tips, food substitutes, and advice on eating out are among the topics covered.

The exercise portion of the program includes games, weight training, and cardiovascular exercise for older children, and balance, coordination, and agility and strength work for younger children. Exercise classes also teach about the effects of exercise on the body.

To help overcome transportation obstacles, the program bought one bus and had another donated. Now, the program can go to the children when the children cannot come to it. To help overcome motivational obstacles, participants receive incentives in the form of T-shirts, water bottles, field trips, and other rewards. Participation is also encouraged by awareness-raising efforts in the local newspapers. School nurses identify potential participants.

The program was funded by a Rural Health Outreach grant from the Office of Rural Health Policy in the Health Resources and Services Administration of the U.S. Department of Health and Human Services and is the product of collaboration between the Ho-Chunk Nation Department of Health, the Ho-Chunk Nation Youth Services Program, the University of Wisconsin-Madison Pediatric Fitness Clinic, three rural school districts, and local pediatricians.

For its innovative efforts, the program received an award from the Pan American Health Organization as part of the 2002 national celebration of World Health Day.

For more information, contact Elliot Blackdeer, Director of the Ho-Chunk Youth Fitness Program, at (715) 284-9851or eblackdeer@ho-chunk.com.

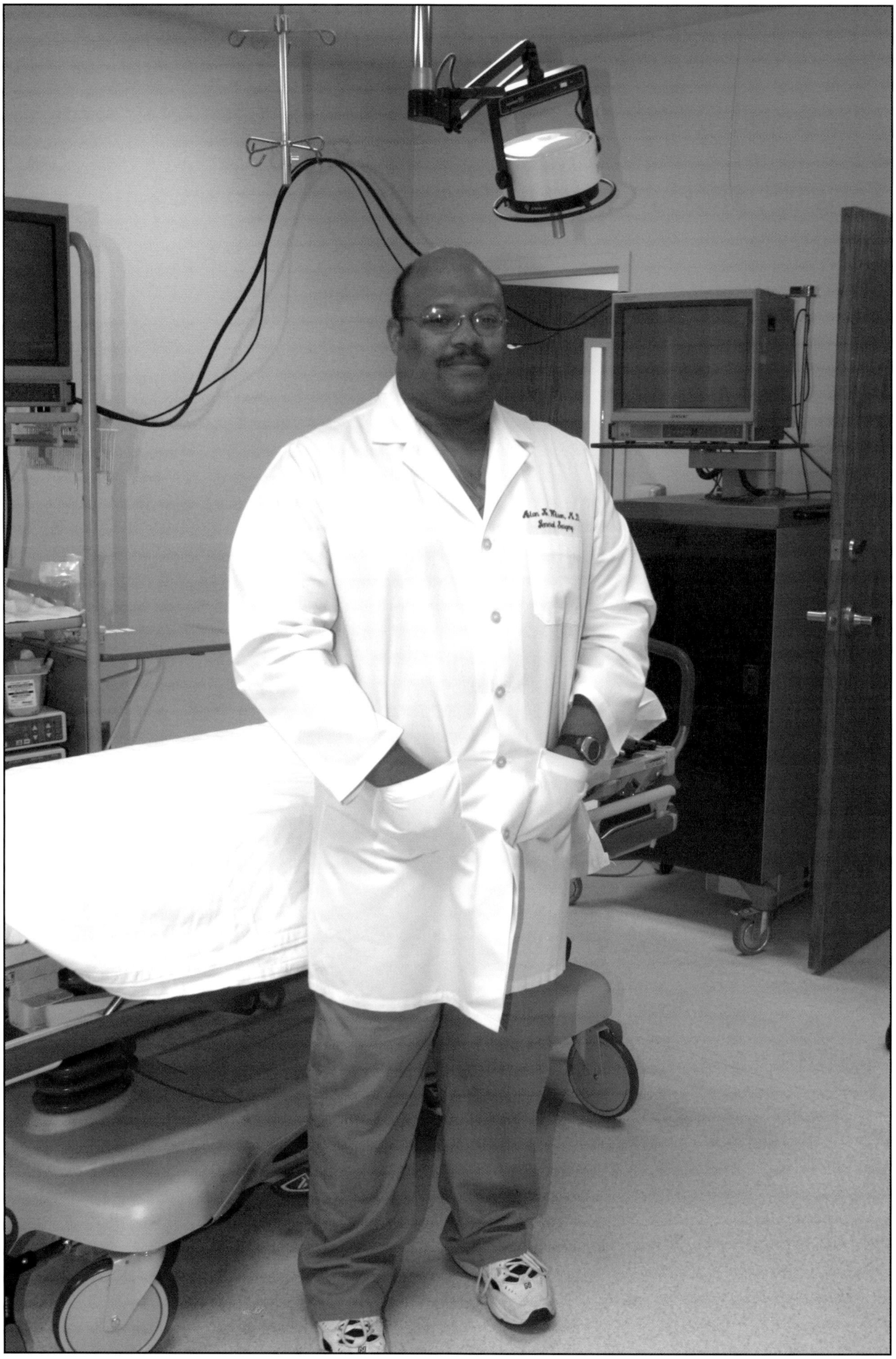

Chapter 4–Improving Facilities

The Challenge

Across the nation, rural hospitals and clinics are aging. Many structures were built in the 1950s with federal monies; many have not been significantly updated since. Why? Often as not, communities simply lack the funds.

As a result of that deterioration, rural health facilities fall farther behind in their ability to provide quality service. The latest medical technology may not be readily available. Physicians, nurses, and technicians may be reticent to practice under such conditions. Even when facilities can provide high-quality service, their age may lead patients to think otherwise and head to the city for treatment.

The Innovations

In Quincy, Illinois, the West Central Illinois Area Agency on Aging scraped together funds from a number of sources to build a new 58,200 square-foot center that has "everything under the sun for seniors"—medical facilities, housing, social activities, job training, and on and on. In all, fourteen separate agencies are located in the building, and 182 groups use it. This innovative co-location means that no one falls through the cracks, and that the whole is far greater than the sum of the parts.

Ashley County, Arkansas, was, until recently, home of one of the last remaining wood-frame hospitals in the country. Not surprisingly, the facility was outdated and obsolete. Since funds to build a new hospital were scarce, however, citizens took it upon themselves to impose a one-cent sales tax to raise the needed money. Once the new facility was built, the hospital was able to recruit new physicians and provide new, previously unavailable, services.

Photo opposite page: Alan Wilson, M.D., in the new Ashley County Memorial Hospital Surgical Unit.

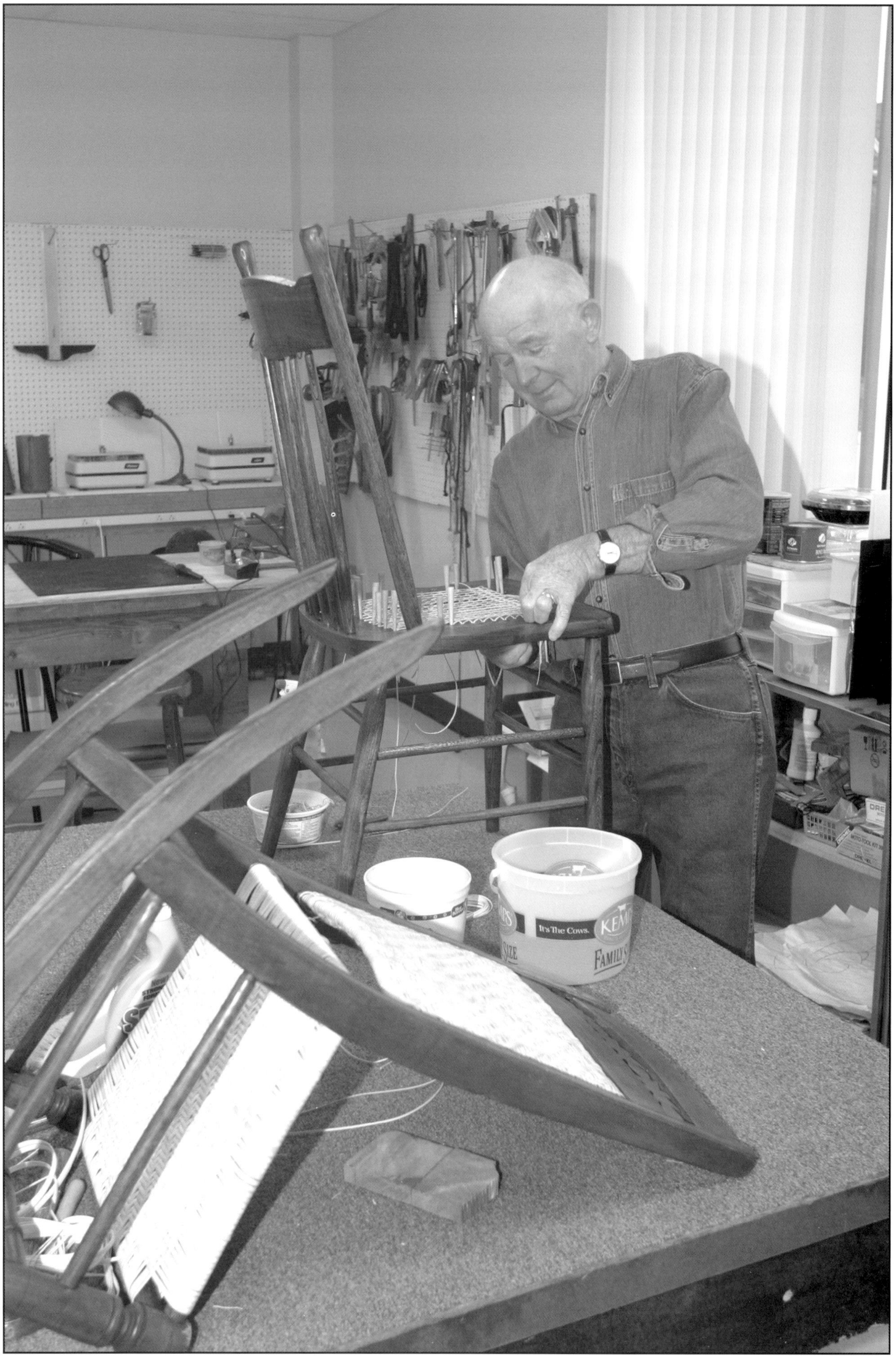
It's The Cows.
FAMILY
SIZE

Giving Seniors Everything, Under One Roof: Quincy Senior and Family Resource Center—Illinois

At half past eight, early-morning craftsmen are caning chairs and chewing the fat in the workshop. Those of a more academic bent have their noses in books in the library. Down the hall, the athletically inclined gather for morning exercise. Outside, vans and cars come and go, dropping more people off to participate, picking up others to run errands. And while the dining room is still full of folks eating breakfast, the buzz in the halls is all about lunch. It's Wednesday. It's fried chicken day. Just a typical morning in a very atypical place.

Indeed, the Quincy Senior and Family Resource Center in Quincy, Illinois, is not your typical rural senior center. First of all, it sits in the middle of downtown, surrounded by a city of 42,000 people. Second, in addition to the workshop, library, exercise rooms, dining hall-cum-ballroom, and a whole host of other amenities, it contains fifty-seven residential apartments; it houses fourteen separate agencies, each offering multiple services to seniors; and it provides meeting and activity space to an astounding 182 groups. All in all, there is nothing typical about it.

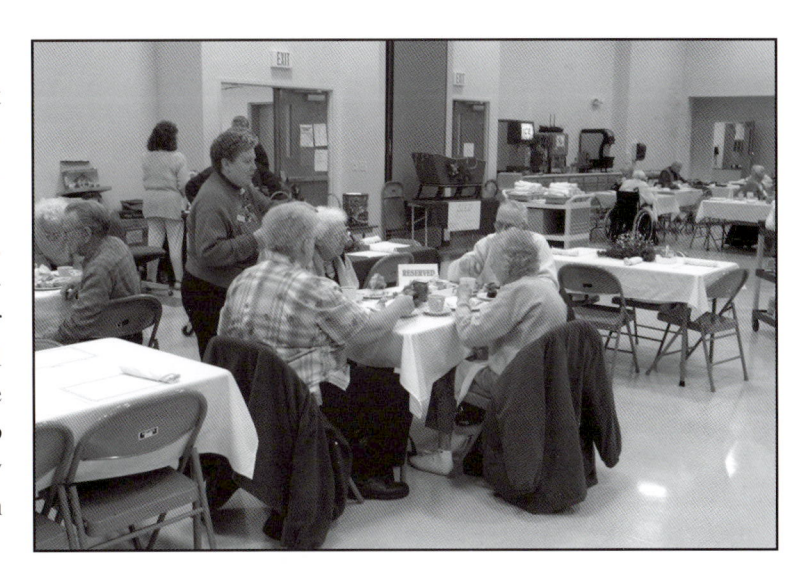

"We're unique in the state, if not the nation," says Lynn Niewohner, Director of the West Central Illinois Area Agency on Aging (WCIAAA), a 501(c)(3) group that owns and operates the facility.

The Program

Opened in December 2002, the center—and the agency—serves a six-county area that stretches across miles of farmland dotted with small

Photos: In addition to the dining hall, above, the center has rooms for hobbies and crafts, such as wood working and chair caning.

towns, thus accounting for its claim as a "rural" center. After Quincy, the next largest town around has only 4,500 people. The agency is the smallest, based on population, of Illinois' thirteen area agencies on aging.

"We're the thirteenth largest," jokes Niewohner.

That said, the agency still serves a population of 25,000 senior citizens. It does that through a wide range of offerings, partnerships, and facilities throughout its service area. The center is just the latest and greatest—and biggest.

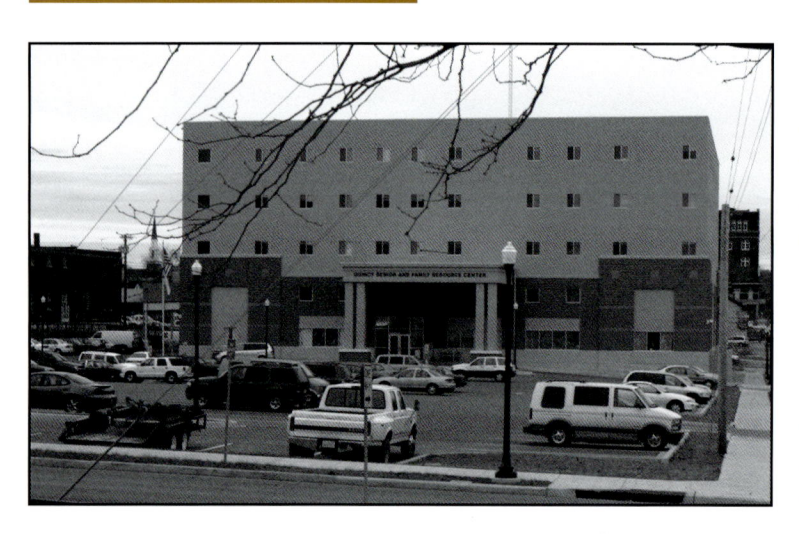

> *. . . nearly 14,000 different seniors come over the course of a year.*

According to Niewohner, 1,000 to 1,500 seniors come through the doors of the four-story, 58,200 square-foot center everyday, double or triple the number that came through the center this one replaced. In all, nearly 14,000 different seniors come over the course of a year.

The reasons they come (and the activities, services, and amenities they find) run the imaginable gamut and then some; everything from simple socializing and adult day care to help with anything from getting a job to overcoming an addiction. A specially trained police officer who deals only with issues pertaining to senior citizens even has an office in the building. Perhaps best of all, the Center hosts a seniors' happy hour every Friday afternoon for friends and family to gather and catch up, with a variety of refreshments available.

"You name it, we've got it," says Niewohner. "Everything under the sun for seniors."

And that, she says, is the beauty of this building. "If we don't combine it all under one roof, it all gets fragmented. Here, you just walk across the hall and see whoever you need to see. No one falls through the cracks."

On top of all the other reasons seniors come to the center, some even come to live.

On the fourth floor are fifty-seven supportive-living apartments for people 65 years and older who need help with the day-to-day activities of life and are at risk of institutionalization. A few are available at market rate ($1900 a month); the rest are for lower-income folks. (In Illinois, supportive living is defined as subsidized assisted living.) With the apartments come meals, help with housekeeping, help with laundry, help with medicines, help with anything that's needed. But the apartments—studios, one- and two-bedrooms—are just that, apartments.

"We're not a nursing home," says Todd Shackelford, WCIAAA Assistant Director. "You'll never see a med cart here. This is not institutional living."

"These are people's homes," says Niewohner.

In one of the apartments, Southern Illinois University (SIU) Medical School runs a health clinic for the supportive-living residents and ultimately for other seniors served by WCIAAA. The clinic is currently open one day a week and staffed by Primary Care Nurse Practitioner Marsha Phillips and Medical Technician Lisa Atwell.

In addition to Phillips and Atwell, a whole team of providers—pharmacist, social worker, physical therapist, occupational therapist, and nutritionist—helps with each of the patients by reviewing his or her situation monthly, as a team, to determine the best course of action. Because center staff often have important information about patients and are right there to talk to Phillips and Atwell, they, too, are considered informally as part of the team and contribute a great deal to the patients' overall care. The result: an interdisciplinary approach to medicine that Phillips says is "the only way to go."

Not just a health care facility, the clinic also serves as a training ground in geriatric medicine for SIU medical residents by bringing them in for rotations and by putting them through an immersion program in geriatric life. In the immersion program, SIU medical residents will, for example, don eyeglasses that distort vision and gloves that limit dexterity and will then be asked to perform tasks such as opening pill bottles, reading pharmaceutical instructions, and the like—things that seniors must do regularly despite debilitating conditions.

The goal, says Phillips, is for the clinic "to be a place where we learn what the geriatric population needs."

"You name it, we've got it. Everything under the sun for seniors."

Lynn Niewohner

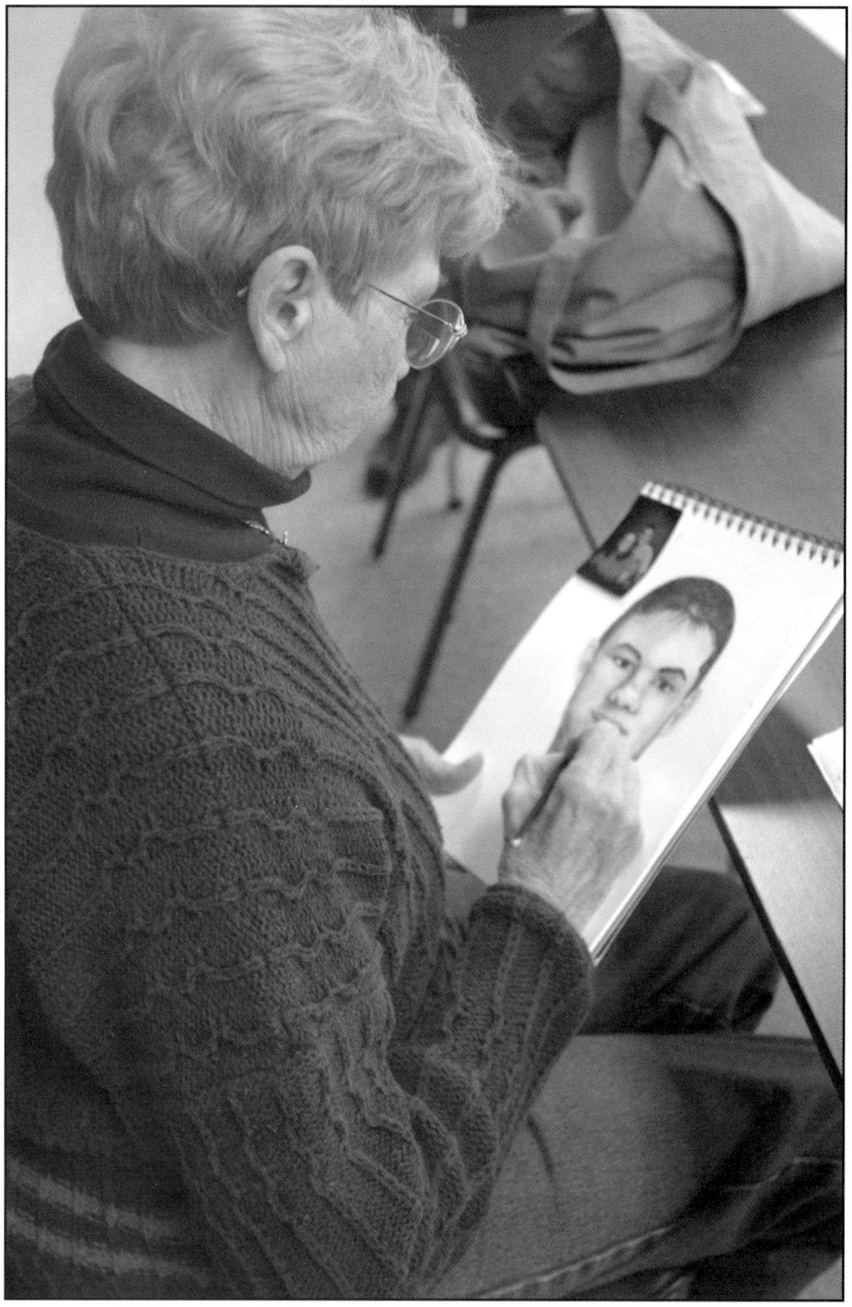

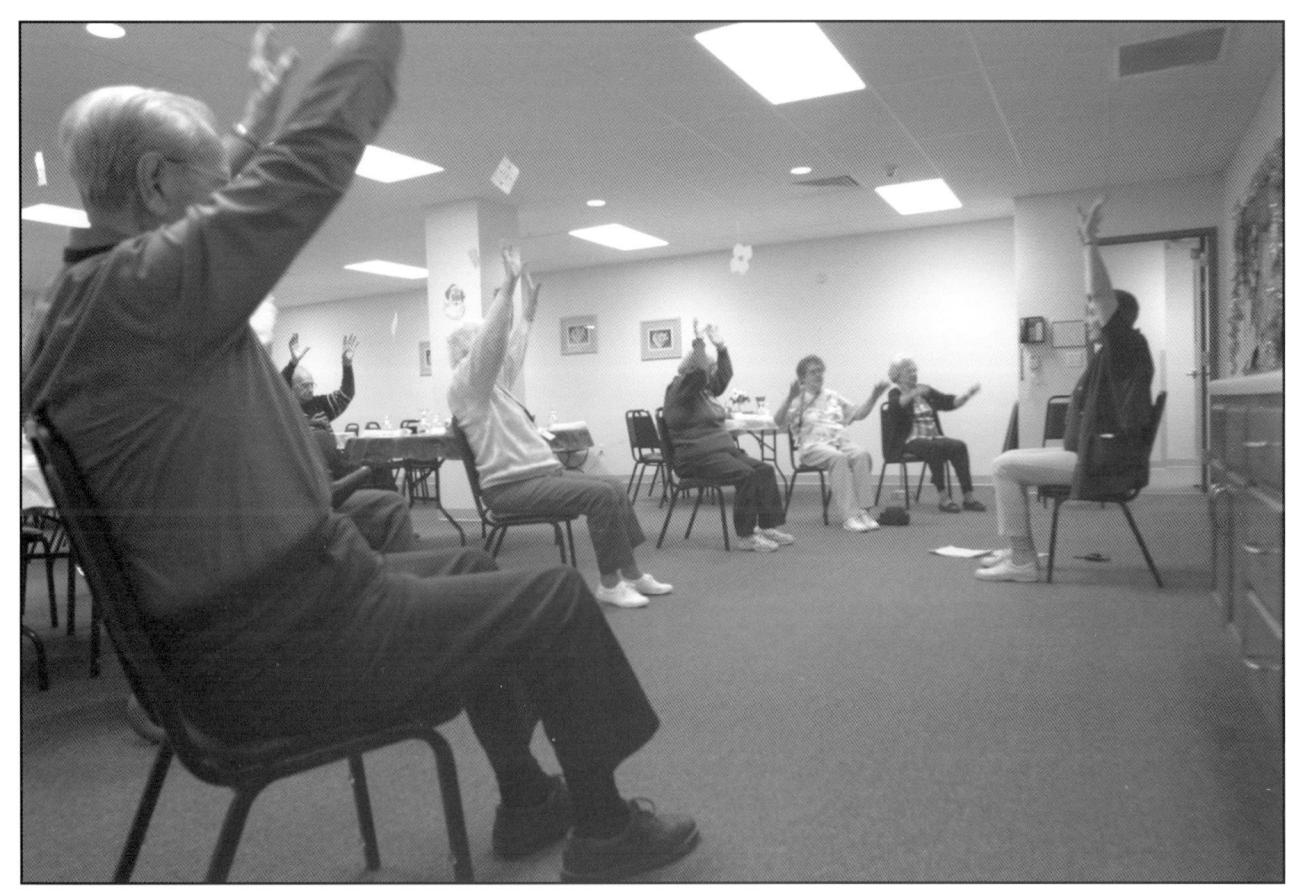

The center's activities also include art and exercise classes.

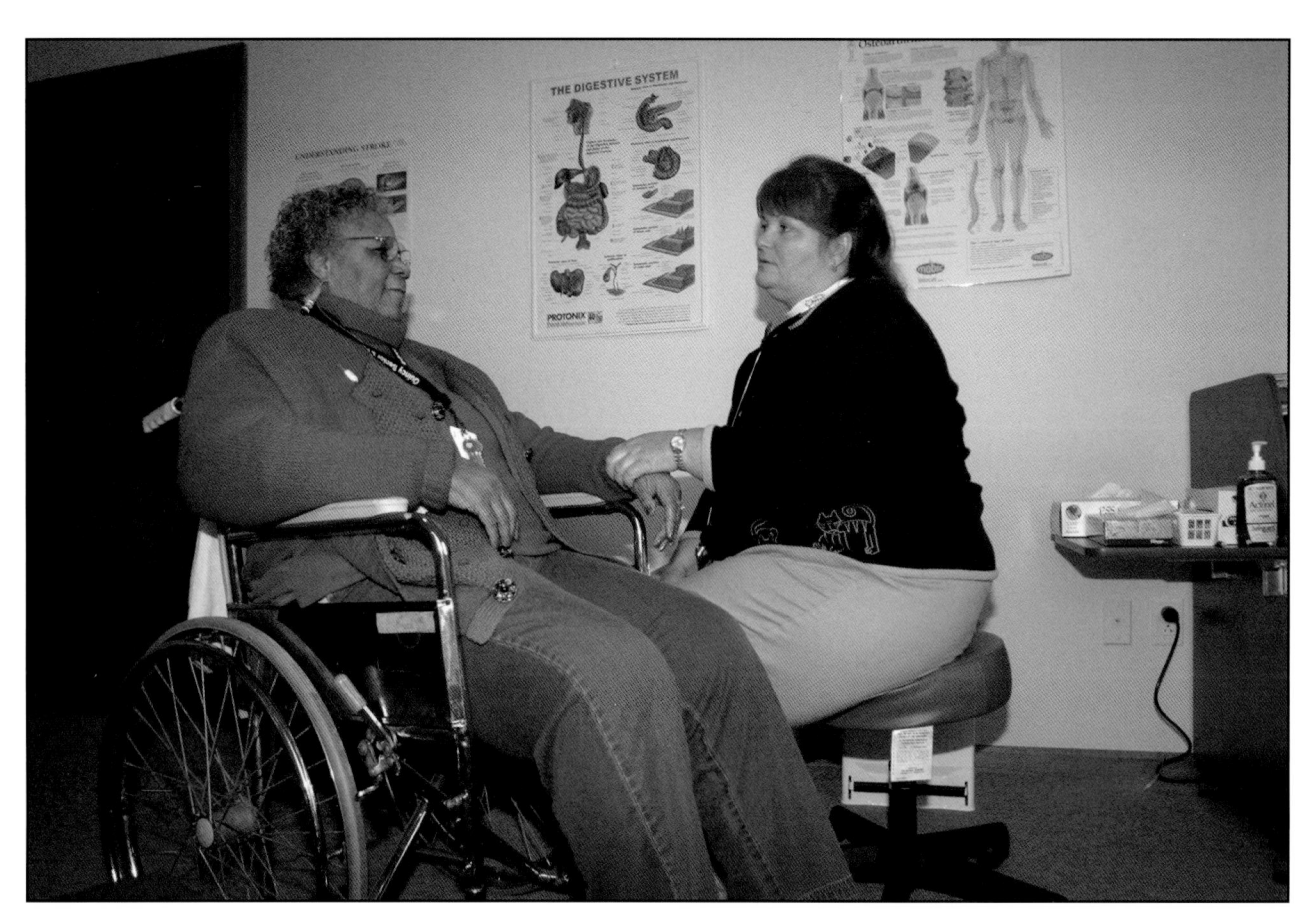

Center resident Ina Bassett with Marsha Phillips, N.P.

The goal of the whole building is to then meet those needs. To help do that, Niewohner and her staff emphasize the rights of seniors and empower them to make decisions about their own lives.

"This business is all about senior citizens," says Niewohner. "What do they want? It's not about us."

That attitude and way of doing business, she says, "came out of our hearts" after seeing how things worked in typical elder institutions. Embodied in the approach are several core values: know each person; put the person before the task; respond to spirit, as well as mind and body; community is the antidote to institutionalization; and all elders are entitled to self-determination wherever they live. All of which, says Niewohner, is "a culture change" from the nursing home business.

"Thirty years in the business," she says, "and I'm scared to death of going to a nursing home."

Results

The co-location of multiple services, combined with an attitude that empowers seniors, results in both efficiency and synergy: the whole is greater than the sum of the parts. That equals better care. And better care means happier, more productive seniors.

Ina Bassett seems to agree. Were it not for the center, Bassett does not know where she would live. The widowed mother of four has arthritis, which keeps her in a wheelchair most of the time. At the moment, she cannot recall her age. What she can recall is that the van that takes her shopping and to church also takes her to visit friends in the nursing home. She doesn't want to end up there.

"This place learns you to do what you need to do, so you're not a dumb-dumb sitting there," says Bassett. "You're well taken care of. You do what you want to. You're not pushed and shoved."

"I love it here," she says with a smile.

According to Phillips, smiles are common. "I've never seen a grumpy face here," she says. "I want to live here."

"I've never seen a grumpy face here. I want to live here."

Marsha Phillips

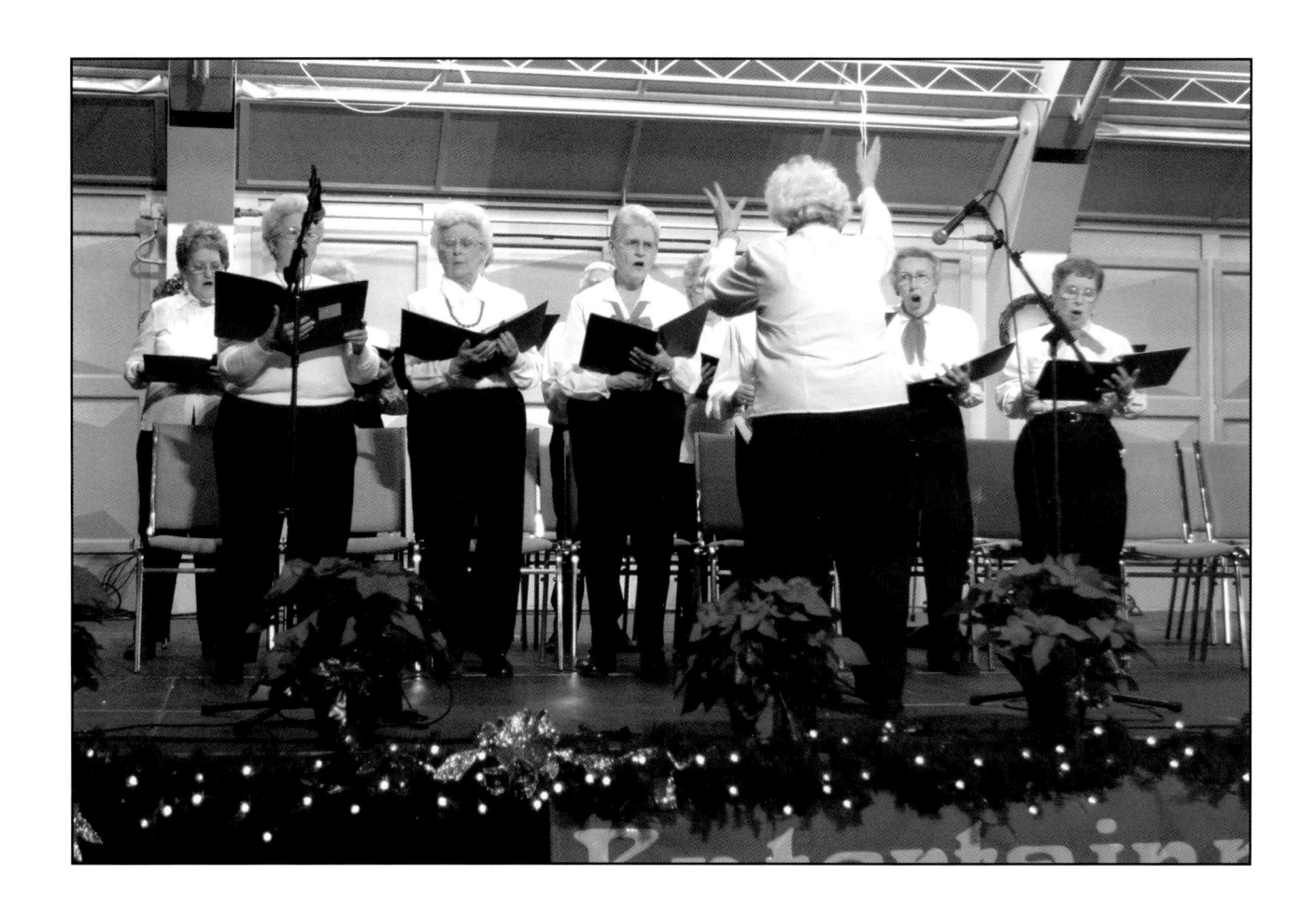

Just the Facts

Purpose

The Quincy Senior and Family Resource Center provides a comprehensive array of services for seniors, including supportive living and health care.

Target Population

The center serves senior citizens in Adams, Brown, Calhoun, Hancock, Pike, and Schuyler counties in west central Illinois.

Partners

The WCIAAA owns and runs the center and shares the facility with fourteen other agencies and 182 groups that serve seniors and families.

Budget

The WCIAAA annual operating budget is $4 million, $300,000 of which is to operate the center. Total cost of the center was $14 million, with funding from a variety of state and federal grants and loans.

Results

Between 1,000 and 1,500 seniors access the facility per day. Some 14,000 different seniors use it over the course of a year.

For more information, contact Lynn Niewohner, Director of WCIAAA, at lynn@wciagingnetwork.org.

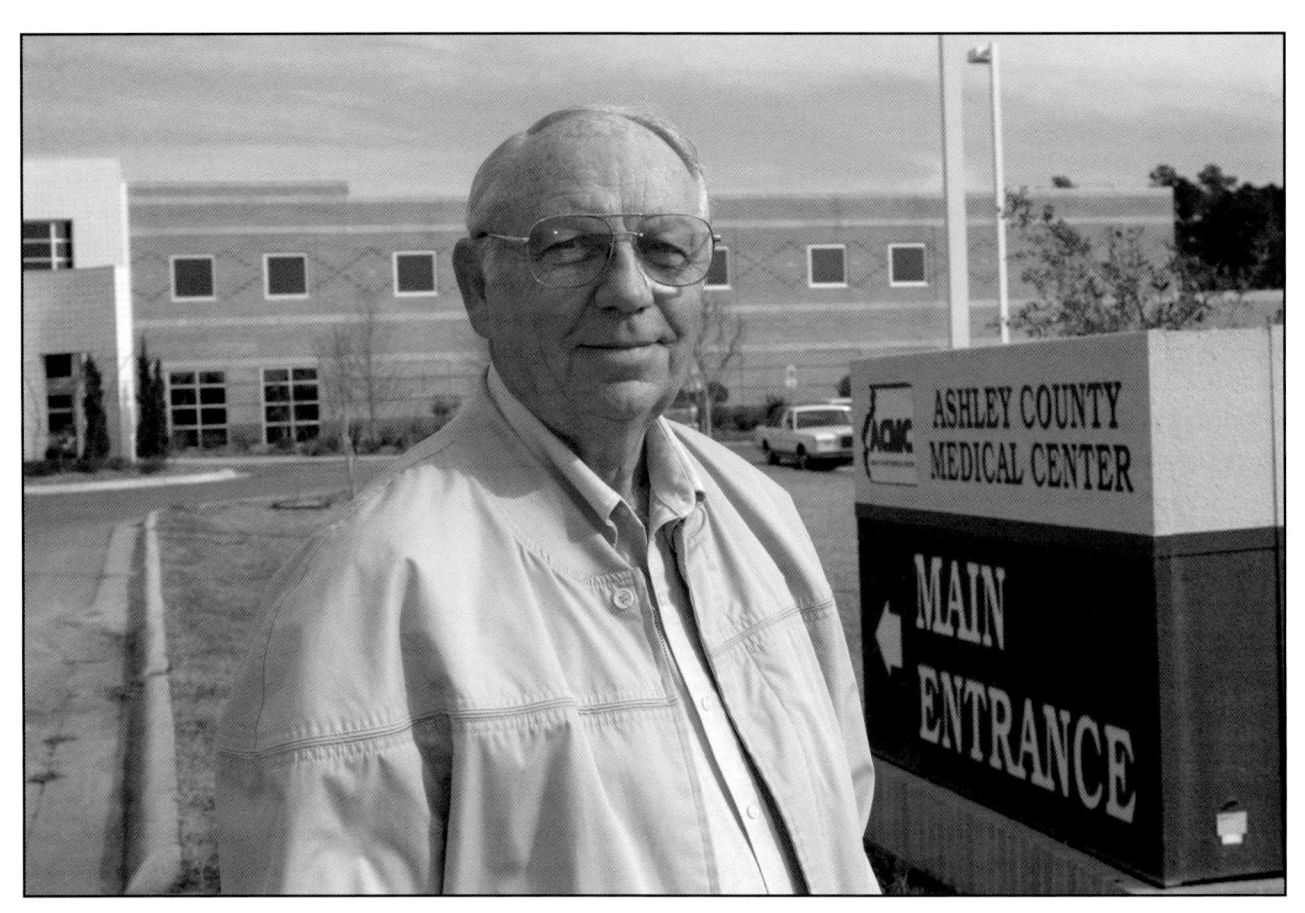

Don Hartley

Raising Taxes, Raising the Standard of Care: Ashley County Medical Center—Arkansas

As one of only two wood-frame hospitals in the nation still in service in the 1990s, Ashley Memorial Hospital in Crossett, Arkansas, was overdue for replacement. In the words of one observer, the structure was "antiquated from one end to the other." Consequently, the community's health care system was at stake, as was its ability to lure and keep residents and businesses, for whom high-quality, local health care is a must.

"The hospital is such a vital function of who we are," says Abby Ebarb, Director of the Crossett Area Chamber of Commerce. "You can't convince a business to come to a town that doesn't take care of the basics. I don't know how we'd function without it."

So in typical fashion for a community that has taxed itself numerous times to improve its quality of life (a new library, a new recreational complex, new streets, and an economic development foundation) the citizens of Ashley County stepped up to the plate and built themselves a new hospital—Ashley County Medical Center.

"When some communities are asking for federal or state help, we look first to ourselves," says Ebarb. "We've always taken care of ourselves."

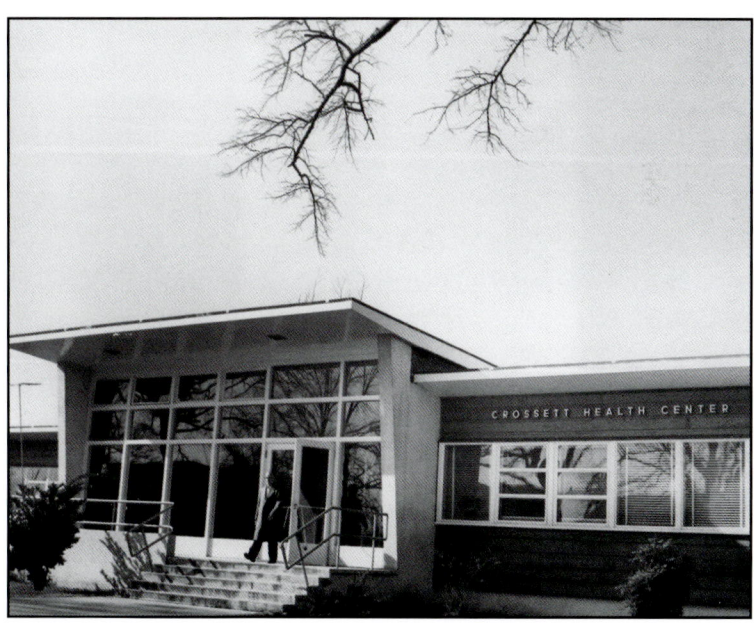

Crossett's old, wood-frame hospital.

"The people in this area are more salt of the earth, hardworking people that don't expect something for nothing," agrees Nancy Foote Spivey, an original member of the new hospital's board. "The people are used to working for what they have and they knew if they wanted this hospital they were going to have to pay for it."

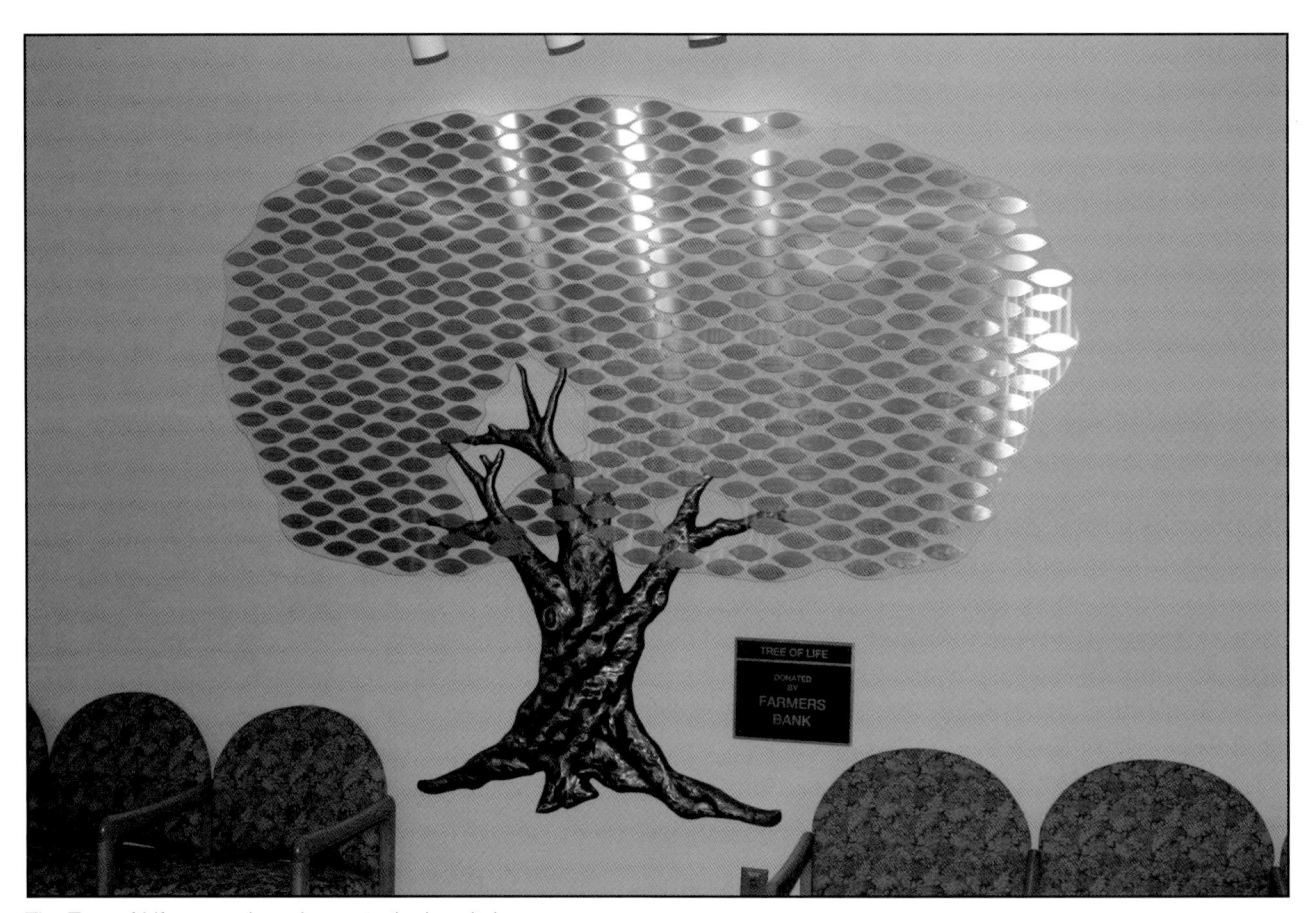

The Tree of Life recognizes donors to the hospital.

And pay for it they did, by floating $12.5 million in municipal bonds and voting in a 1 percent county sales tax to pay them off.

The Program

Favorable though the outcome, the road to it was neither short nor straight.

The old hospital, built in the 1950s, was owned and operated by a nonprofit organization. It had long needed help. Not only was the facility outdated, it was also too large, designed for a time when in-patient services far exceeded outpatient services. Consequently, it was also underutilized and expensive to run. To top it all off, certain basic services were not available.

"The old hospital had gotten the reputation of being a glorified band-aid station—no babies, no broken bones," says Pam Ferguson, director of Marketing and Public Relations at Ashley County Medical Center (ACMC). Getting such care meant driving forty-five miles to the next closest in-state hospital.

In light of the hospital's troubles, the hospital board came up with a plan for a new hospital, to be owned by the county, run by a county-appointed board, and funded by a sales tax increase. That, however, meant approval first from the county's quorum court (the county's legislative body) and second from voters. The court agreed and County Judge Don Hartley, Ashley County's chief administrative official, went to work promoting the new hospital and the sales tax at public events, on the radio, and in the local newspapers.

In March 1994, the sales tax passed by a vote of three to one.

"The people of Ashley County were very much in favor of building a new hospital," says Spivey, "because they knew that was the only way we could have good health care locally."

"I'm not a politician, never was," says Hartley. "I always wanted to get the job done."

According to Spivey, Hartley is indeed the one who got the job done. "We felt like this hospital should have the name Ashley County on it because the citizens, the voters, they're the ones that ultimately paid for

"The people are used to working for what they have and they knew if they wanted this hospital they were going to have to pay for it."

Nancy Foote Spivey

> *"My feeling was the [new] hospital was not overstaffed, it was underutilized. What we had to do was increase our utilization."*
>
> Russ Sword

it and it is everyone's facility. So it shouldn't have a person's name, but if there had been a person it would have been Don Hartley. He championed the cause. It would never have happened without him."

Hartley's involvement, however, did not stop after the vote. As chief administrative officer of the county, he appointed the new hospital board, a task he says was the most difficult of his career. He also oversaw the bidding and construction of the hospital, oftentimes saving money by using county work crews and even inmates from a nearby prison.

"A lot of work went into this thing to get it ready," he says.

The new hospital opened in June 1998, but that's still only half the story.

Russ Sword arrived in December 1998 as interim CEO of the hospital. His task was to keep things running while finding a permanent chief. What he found was a gleaming new facility, yet one in dire financial straits.

With eleven doctors on staff and expenses exceeding revenue, the board believed that the hospital was overstaffed. Sword, a veteran of starting and reviving small rural hospitals around the country, saw it differently.

"My feeling was the hospital was not overstaffed, it was underutilized," he says. "What we had to do was increase our utilization."

To do that meant recruiting new doctors as well as different kinds of doctors. At the time, nine of the eleven doctors on staff were primary care physicians. Sword wanted more specialists.

According to Sword, primary care has been pushed upon rural areas, yet it is extremely difficult for a hospital to succeed solely as a primary care facility. The reason: most primary care doctors today do not utilize hospitals.

"Primary care doctors think it's a failure on their part if their patients have to go to a hospital," he says. "They practice outpatient care and refer to a specialist if the patients need to go into a hospital. Hospitals without specialists don't get the business and they can't carry their overhead."

Sword went in search of specialists and landed several: an obstetrician, an orthopedic surgeon, a pulmonologist, and an oncologist. Two of the specialists are also so-called hospitalists, doctors who practice only inpatient medicine. Their presence on staff gives the hospital a way to get referrals and thus increase business. On advice from the Rural Hospital Performance Improvement Project, an assistance program of the Office of Rural Health Policy, Sword is helping pay for the hospitalists by also assigning them to cover the emergency department half time.

Emmanuel Bayongan, M.D., in the United States on a J-1 visa waiver, is one of the hospitalists. Bayongan says he interviewed at five different hospitals before choosing Ashley County. He liked what he saw: a place to practice his specialty, pulmonology, and a pace that would not burn him out.

"They made it very very convenient for me to move down here," says the 35-year-old doctor from the Philippines who trained in New York. "This place was the best place that I could find. I'm planning to stay."

Alan Wilson, M.D., is the hospital's and the county's lone general surgeon. He practiced briefly at the old facility.

"If it was cold, it was cold; if it was hot, it was hot," Wilson says of the old building. "A lot of people had misgivings with the older hospital."

The new hospital, he says, offered a new beginning and was, in fact, instrumental in his move to Crossett. "Actually, the new hospital is one of the reasons why I'm here. When I was recruited they said we're building a new hospital and I said 'well that would be neat.'"

In addition to adding doctors, ACMC has added specialty outpatient services and built a provider-based Rural Health Clinic next door to capture business that would otherwise go elsewhere. The hospital has also subdivided its property and sold and developed lots to generate revenue and attract other medical providers. Finally, Sword and his staff are actively engaged in the life of the community, participating in economic development efforts, hosting community events, and serving on the Chamber of Commerce.

"I think that's critically important, for the hospital to be a part of the community and to be active in the community," says Sword. "We do everything we can to make sure we are visible."

"Actually, the new hospital is one of the reasons why I'm here."

Alan Wilson

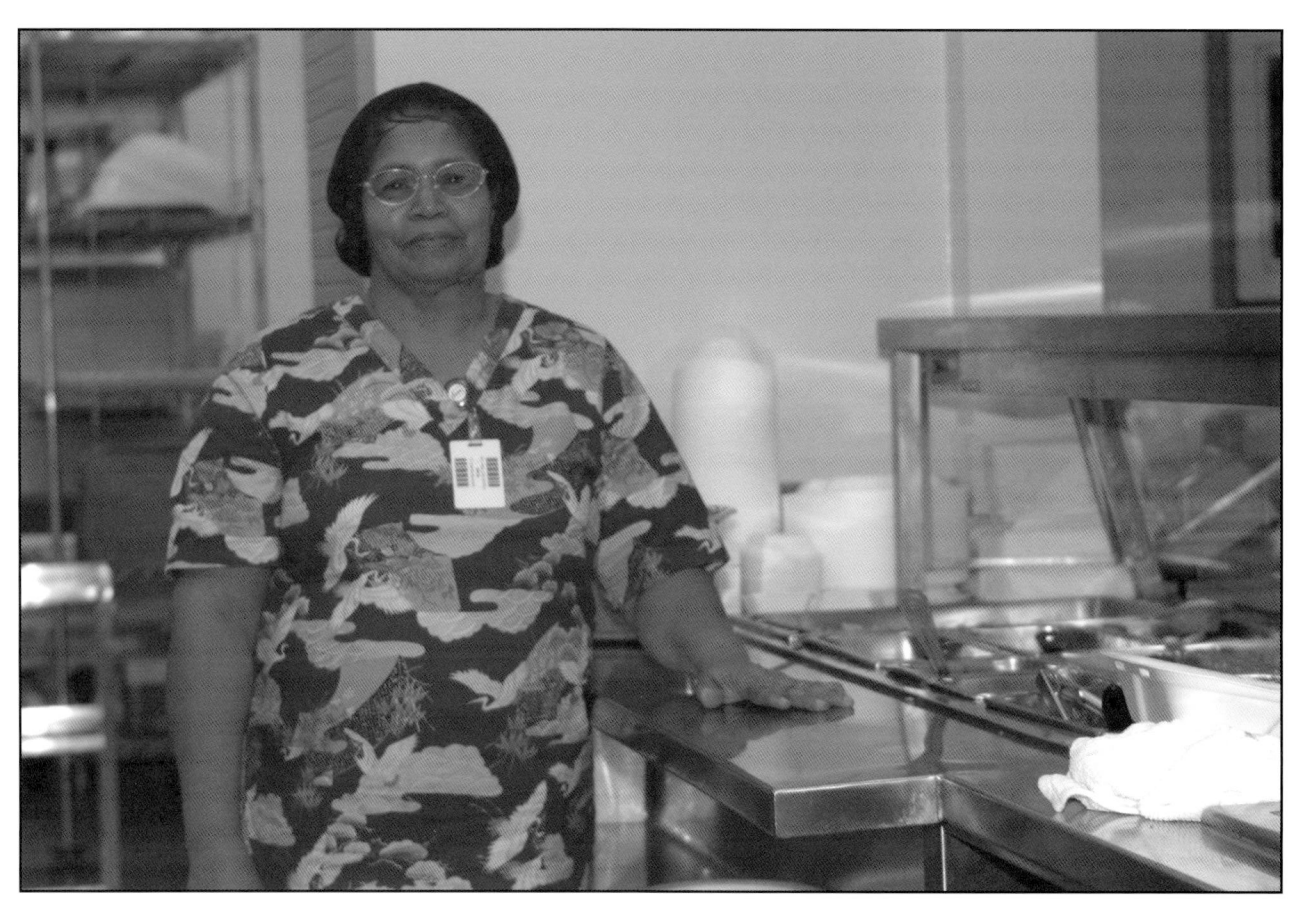

Veteran of the old facility, Mary Childress prefers the new.

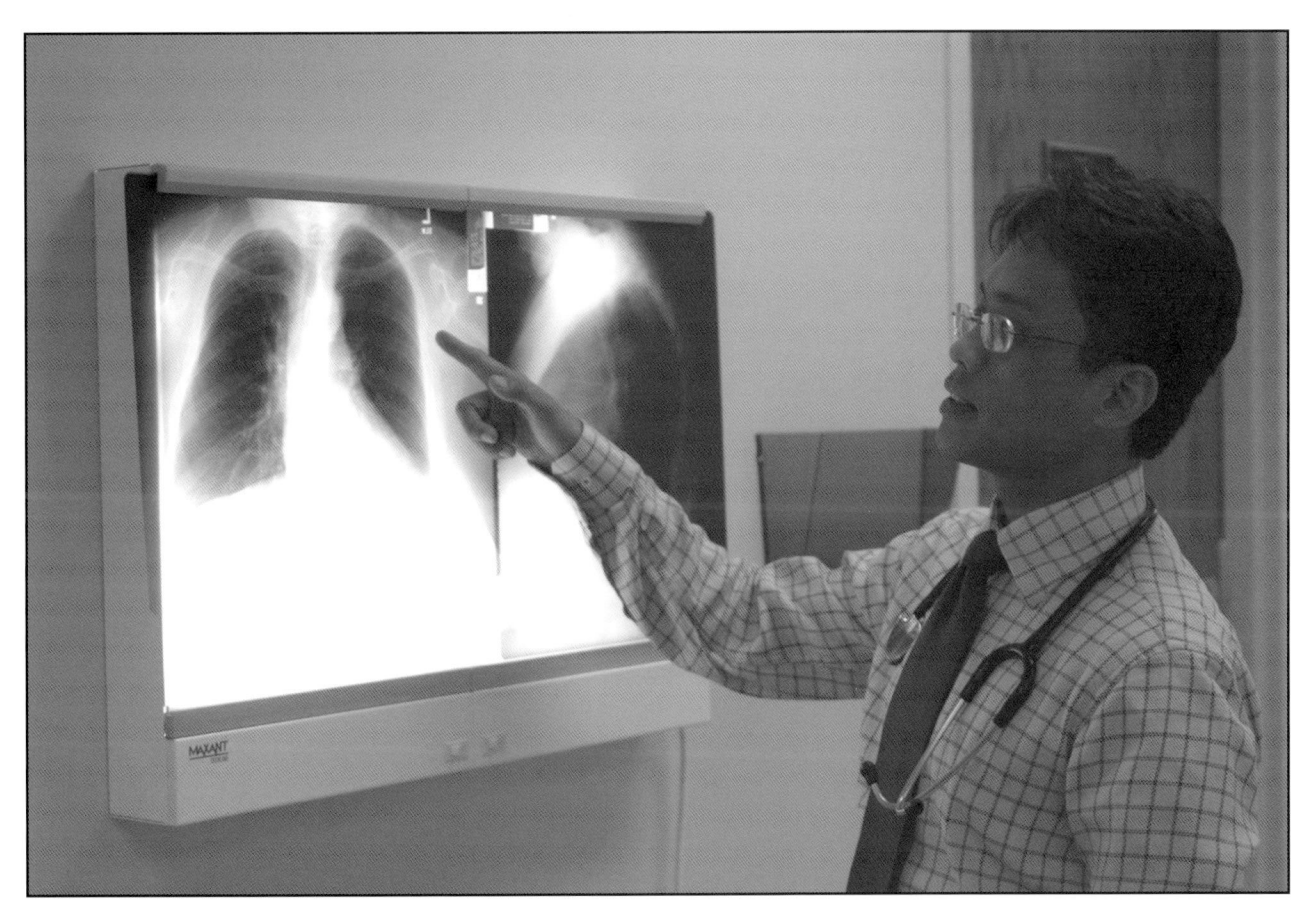

Emmanuel Bayongan, M.D.

Results

Through all its efforts, ACMC has improved the area's health care and, by extension, its economic potential. Outpatient services are up. New doctors are on board.

That success notwithstanding, the hospital's financial future is still a bit uncertain. Sword figures that to be economically sustainable, the hospital must increase its overall utilization by five inpatients per day. Whether it can achieve that, it's too early to tell. The new doctors have just come on board. So, for now, the hospital is making it "from paycheck to paycheck" while doing all that it can to get the hospital on firm financial ground.

"We enjoy small-town life," he says, "but we also know that you have to grow to continue to survive." He is confident that growth will come, if given enough time.

If Don Hartley is concerned about the future, he doesn't let on. "It's one of the best things that ever happened to Ashley County. In my opinion, this is one of the finest small facilities in the country."

"It's been like a dream come true," says Spivey.

> *"It's one of the best things that ever happened to Ashley County. In my opinion, this is one of the finest small facilities in the country."*
>
> Don Hartley

Just the Facts

Purpose

Ashley County Medical Center is a county-owned facility leased to and run by a nonprofit organization. Its mission: to provide comprehensive health care to area residents.

Target Population

The hospital serves residents of Ashley County, Arkansas, and the surrounding region.

Partners

The Medical Center was made possible by a 1 percent county-wide sales tax passed by county voters, a gift of land by the Georgia-Pacific Company, and donations by citizens and businesses.

Budget

The facility cost $12.5 million to build and equip. Total annual expenses are approximately $16.8 million.

Results

In 2003, the hospital had 17,074 patient visits and gross revenue of $13,746,773. Outpatient services have increased some 25 percent since the move. The new facility also made possible recruitment of five new specialists, one each in obstetrics/gynecology, internal medicine, pulmonology/critical care, oncology/hematology, and orthopedic surgery.

For more information, contact Pam Ferguson, Director of Marketing and Public Relations, at pferguson@acmconline.org.

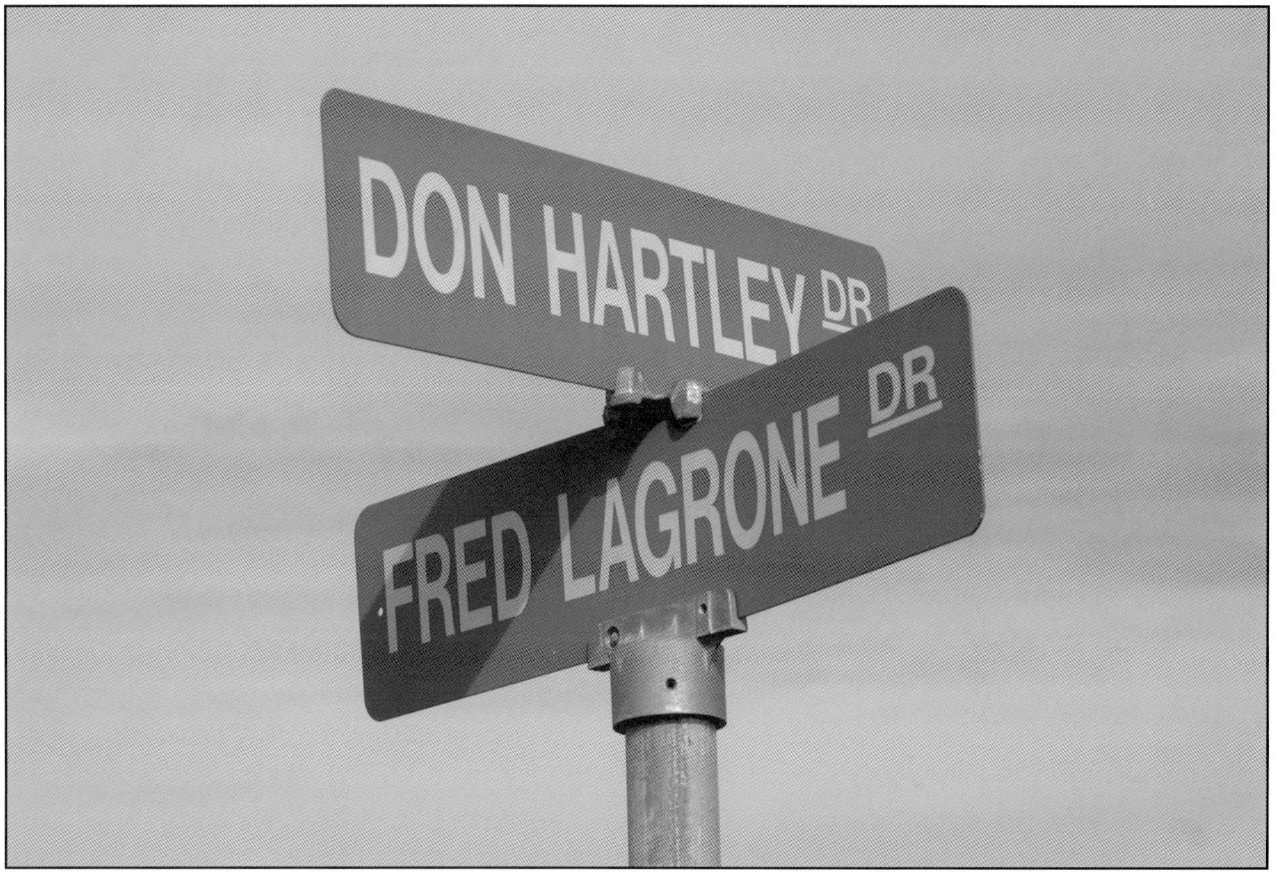
DON HARTLEY DR
FRED LAGRONE DR

Building Hospitals:
HUD 242 Program—Colorado and Idaho

Coming up with funds to improve or replace aging or inadequate rural medical facilities is all too often akin to finding the proverbial needle in the haystack. A new twist on an old program, however, is helping to change that.

The U.S. Department of Housing and Urban Development (HUD) has streamlined its Federal Housing Administration 242 Hospital Insurance program to make it easier for Critical Access Hospitals (CAHs) to participate. Now, CAHs can get loan guarantees to help finance construction, and modernization efforts.

The 242 program enhances a borrower's creditworthiness by insuring the mortgage and taking the risk out of lending. Consequently, loans are easier to come by and at better rates. As such, the program will provide Critical Access Hospitals with better access to much-needed capital. Prior to streamlining, the program had focused almost entirely on urban hospitals.

According to Betty Kavanaugh, Vice President of PNC Multifamily Capital, an FHA-approved lender, the mortgage insurance can be utilized by an FHA lender to provide financing on a taxable basis or as credit enhancement for tax-exempt bonds. The enhancement effectively gives a hospital an AA rating and allows it to get a higher loan amount than most conventional options.

In May 2003, HUD announced the first-ever insurance commitments for CAHs: Rio Grande Hospital in Del Norte, Colorado, and Shoshone Medical Center in Kellogg, Idaho.

In Del Norte, a town of 1,709 residents located in the San Luis Valley of south central Colorado, the insurance will enable the much-needed replacement of a 50-year-old facility. The new hospital, scheduled to open in July 2004, will have fourteen beds, an expanded emergency department, and space for laboratory, physical therapy, pharmacy, and administration functions. The 242 program will insure $10 million of the $11.5 million cost of the project. Rio Grande worked with Kavanaugh's firm on the deal.

The Shoshone Medical Center in the northern Idaho town of Kellogg will be a $20.5 million twenty-five-bed replacement facility serving as the principal health care provider for Shoshone County, a mountainous region of 2,640 square miles with a population of approximately 15,000. The new facility, which will open in November 2004, will include a permanent magnetic resonance imaging unit, a breast cancer screening unit, and expanded outpatient diagnostic and surgical services. The program will insure $18.5 million of the total cost of the project.

The old facility, says CEO Gary Moore, was shot, and repairing it would have cost more than building a new facility. Still, funding for a new facility was hard to come by. "We wouldn't be building the new hospital if it wasn't for the 242," he says. "No commercial lender would look at us. They consider small rural hospitals just too risky."

Norman Haug, M.D., administrator at Rio Grande concurs. "Without the HUD 242 program, we'd have a difficult time finding funding," says Haug. "We're a nonprofit hospital in a relatively poor area with a high Medicare population. We're too high of a risk for most lenders."

The program has made a believer out of Moore. "I tell other rural hospital administrators to go and find their financing, and when they can't, to look to the 242."

"I think it's the appropriate way to go for a small rural hospital," says Haug.

For more information, contact Moore at (208) 786-0581, Haug at (719) 657-2510, or Kavanaugh at (678) 624-3099, betty.kavanaugh@pnc.com.

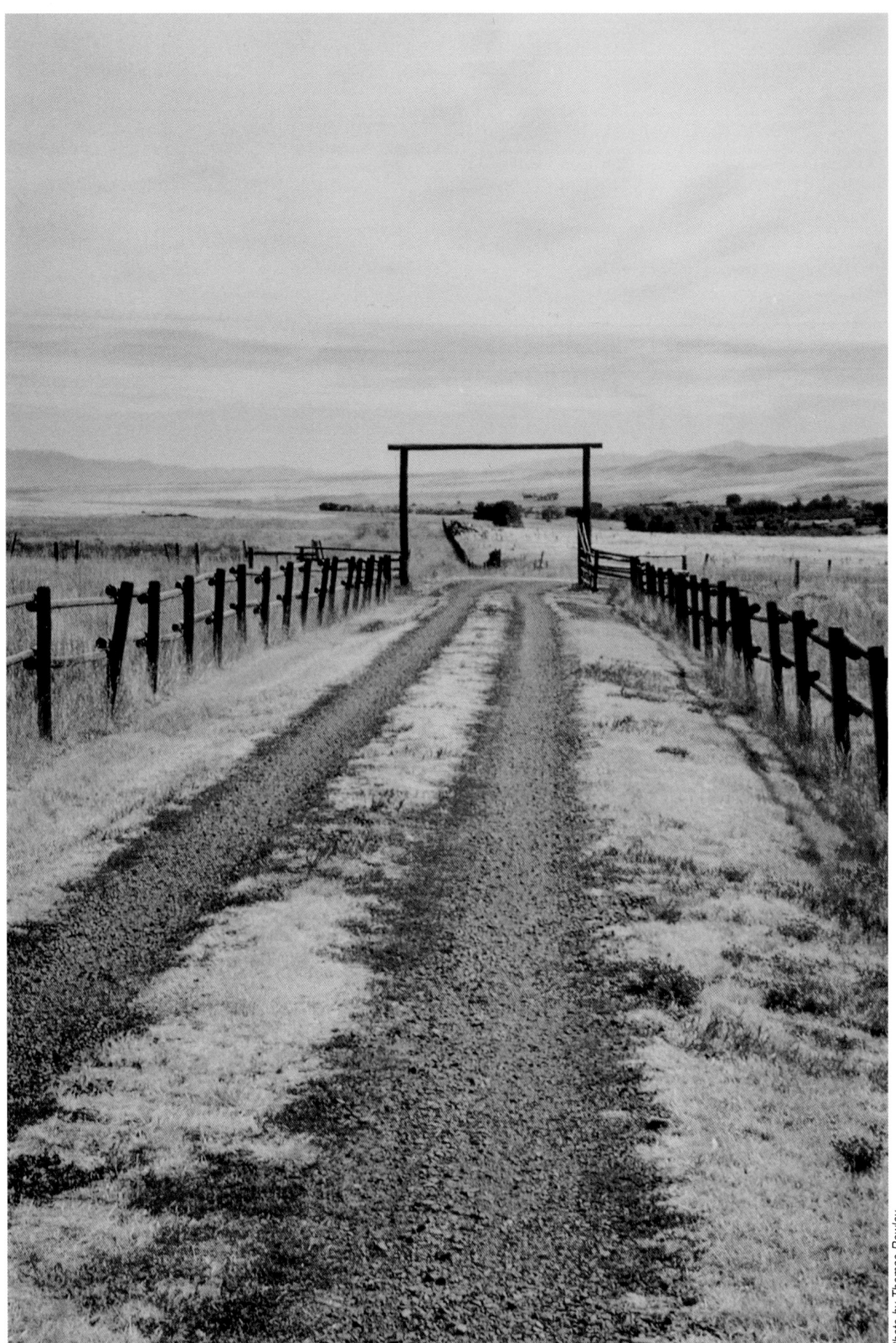

Photo by Thomas Rowley

Chapter 5–Reaching the Remote

The Challenge

Many challenges to rural health care stem from the very characteristics of rural life. Sparse population density, long distances, and lagging economies make it both physically and financially difficult to reach and serve the people living there. In truly remote rural areas—areas far removed from population centers, often by difficult terrain as well as by sheer distance, where population density is sometimes measured in square miles per person rather than the other way around—these challenges only multiply.

Not surprisingly, health care in remote rural areas often leaves much to be desired. According to the Frontier Education Center in Santa Fe, New Mexico, the majority of the 814 so-called "frontier counties" in the United States have two or fewer health care services of any kind. Seventy-eight frontier counties have no health care services whatsoever. Yet, these counties, spread across 21 states, are home to nearly a quarter of a million people. On much of the frontier, the nearest medical help can be an hour or more away, sometimes much more.

The Innovations

Fortunately, new ideas, techniques, and technologies are helping combat the challenges of remoteness. Using everything from circuit-riding providers to cooperatives to telecommunications linkages, people are finding ways to get the health care they need and deserve, even in the most remote reaches of the country.

In Montana and surrounding states, a project called Women to Women uses the Internet to link together women who live in remote rural areas and have chronic illness. This "virtual support group" provides participants with critical emotional and educational support as they deal with the dual isolation imposed by their geography and their health.

In tiny Condon, Oregon, enterprising residents who were tired of living without local health care created a unique local taxing structure to pay for their very own clinic and medical staff. As a result, this town of 759 people now has round-the-clock care, in a region considered both a Medically Underserved Area and a Health Professional Shortage Area. Through innovations like these, the challenges of remoteness can be met and the people in remote rural America can be served.

Photo opposite page:
Ranch road, Pony, Montana

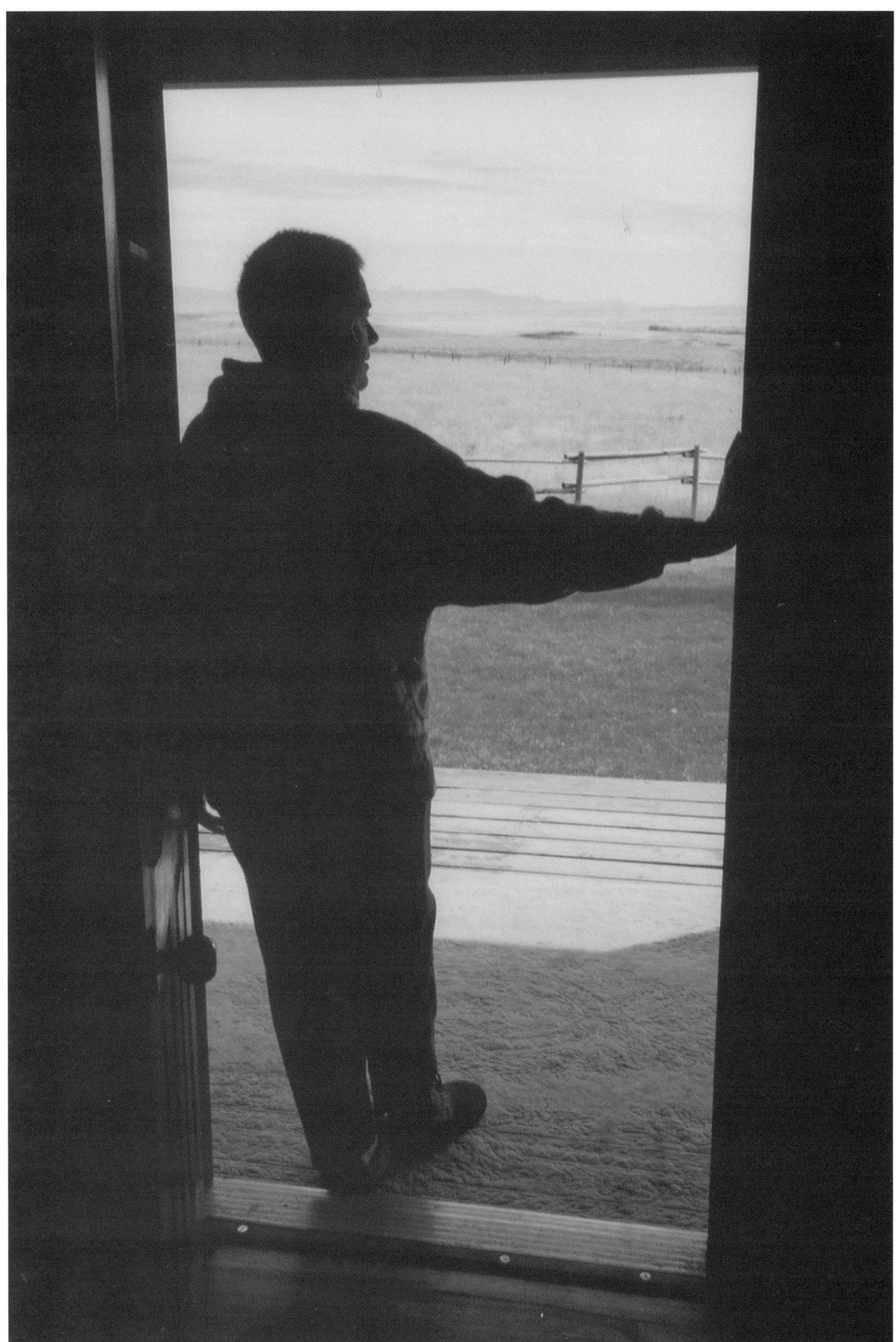

Photos by Thomas Rowley

Connecting and Supporting Chronically Ill Women: Women to Women—Montana and Surrounding States

The view from Nina Sperandeo's front porch is spectacular: mountains, fields, and the Morgan horses she keeps. The scene, however, is telling. Isolation, geographic and otherwise, is a constant in her life.

Pony, Montana, which has been Sperandeo's home for the past seven years, has, she says, "105 mailboxes, 80 year-round residents, and 150 or so in the summer." To reach her, just head west from the two-lane highway a dozen or so miles, turn right onto a street with no sign, and go past the cows. Honk if the dog is in the yard. Getting to there or from there isn't complicated, but for a person with multiple sclerosis, it isn't exactly easy. The closest ambulance is thirty minutes away. The hospital is an hour over the mountain, a drive she describes as a "real bugger" in wind or winter. And her neurologist, who she sees three times a year, is in Great Falls, a good four-hour drive away.

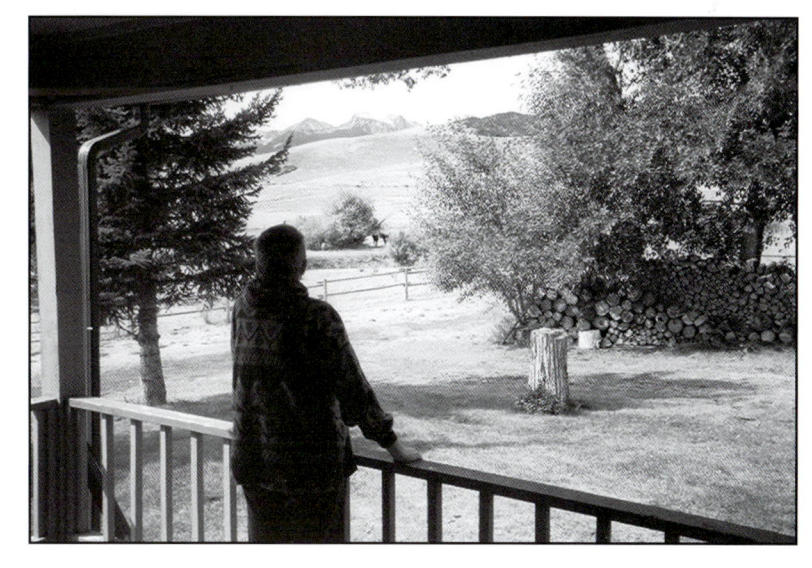

"When there's nobody living near you and you can't see another house…and you're a transplanted city girl, the depression can be overwhelming," says Sperandeo.

Geography, however, isn't Sperandeo's only jailer. Like many people with chronic health conditions, she also suffers the isolation of her illness: not being able to fully participate in many of life's activities, not wanting to burden friends and family, and not having peers who truly understand what one is going through. All of which is made worse by her physical location.

Indeed, combining remoteness and chronic illness makes for an isolation

Photo opposite page and above:
Nina Sperandeo

double-whammy. Diagnosed with MS in 1987, Sperandeo has since gone on Medicare disability, been in and out of a wheelchair, spent a year in bed, been snowed in for weeks, been unable at times to get needed treatments, had a nervous breakdown, and considered suicide.

She also enrolled in Women to Women.

"I wouldn't be here," she says. "I can honestly say that I would not be here if it hadn't been for Women to Women."

Tears in her eyes emphasize the statement.

The Program

Women to Women is the brainchild of Clarann Weinert, Ph.D., a Sister of Charity nurse-sociologist, and Director of the Center for Research on Chronic Health Conditions in Rural Dwellers at the Montana State University-Bozeman, College of Nursing. The program's goal (and Weinert's personal goal) is to "to teach women how to take care of themselves and to live healthier lives despite their chronic health condition." Women to Women does that by offering participants access to both peers and to health education.

Technically, Women to Women is a research project, a way to evaluate telecommunications-enabled (or virtual) support groups for women with chronic conditions in remote areas. It is, however, a research project that provides invaluable service to the study's participants.

The program began in 1996 out of a convergence of Weinert's years of work on rural issues and the mid-1990s boom in telecommunications technology. Her studies kept showing Weinert the importance of social support for people with chronic illness. The technology showed her a way to overcome geographic obstacles and get that support to people who desperately need it.

"We know that small support groups work," says Weinert, citing Alcoholics Anonymous and groups for people with other diseases. "But in rural areas they don't work as well because people are not going to drive a long way, or there are not enough people in the community to do it, or it's snowing, or whatever."

"I wouldn't be here. I can honestly say that I would not be here if it hadn't been for Women to Women."

Nina Sperandeo

The Internet, thought Weinert, could change that. "It's a perfect match for rural," she says.

And that makes it a perfect match for Montana.

With 145,556 square miles of land, Montana is the fourth largest state. With only 6.2 persons per square mile and 275 towns and cities (some 50 percent unincorporated and 80 percent with fewer than 3,000 people), it is also one of the most rural and remote states. On top of that, Montana, like many rural states, has relatively few health care providers. All in all, it seemed the perfect place to try to create virtual support groups. So Weinert—with the help of the Burns Telecommunications Center at Montana State University-Bozeman and funding from twelve different entities, including the Sisters of Charity Ministry Foundation and the National Institutes of Health/National Institute of Nursing Research— did just that.

In rural areas, support groups don't work as well. The Internet could change that.

The concept is straightforward. Recruit women with chronic conditions from rural Montana (and now Idaho, Wyoming, and the Dakotas) to participate. Hook them up to the Internet (providing them with a computer and Internet service if necessary). Train them in the use of the technology. And give them access to e-mail and an electronic chat room where they can interact with one another. The women are also provided with health educational materials on women's health, nutrition, chronic illness, and financial management, and are asked to work their way through it in a certain time frame.

The program enlists women in cohorts, which run for two years (the computer portion lasts twenty-two weeks). Cohorts are staggered so as to maximize the use of equipment. Therefore, three cohorts are running at any one time.

Throughout the program, a nurse monitor and a technical assistance person are available to answer questions and make sure the program stays on course. Evaluation questionnaires are distributed six times over the course of the two years to gauge the women's progress. Other than that, the women are on their own, but now as a caring group of peers, not as isolated individuals.

As that caring group of peers, the women share their experiences with one another: their triumphs and travails, what has worked for them and

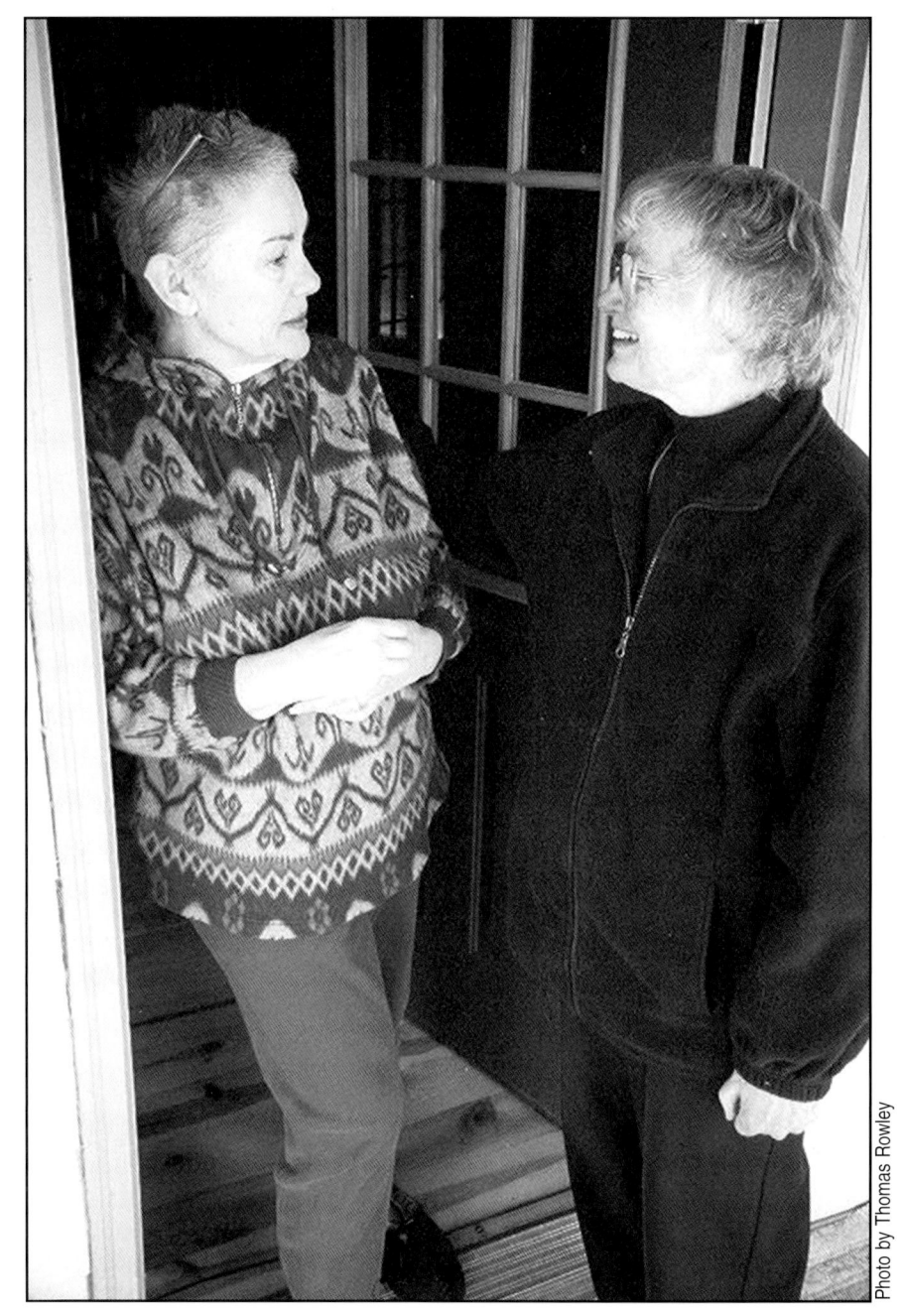

Nina Sperandeo and Women to Women's Shirley Cudney, R.N.

Photo by Thomas Rowley

what has not. They also point each other to helpful websites, research findings, and so on. Perhaps most importantly, they give each other the sympathizing ear and encouraging word that only people who share a common burden can give.

"The things they tell us and each other are just absolutely revelatory," says Weinert. "Some of it is extremely intimate, extremely personal." And that, she says, makes it all the more effective.

"I like that connection," says Sperandeo. "I like that reason to turn on the computer, to get online. To know somebody will be there ... somebody there you can talk to ... somebody to say 'call your doctor, go to the hospital.' Somebody to say 'yeah, I've been there too and this is what I did.' It's like someone validating [what you're going through]. It's both encouragement and the information. If you're up and crying at one o'clock in the morning, you're not going to call your doctor."

"I like that reason to turn on the computer, to get online. To know somebody will be there ... somebody there you can talk to ... ."

Nina Sperandeo

Now in its third two-year iteration, Women to Women involves a cohort of sixty women at a time. To participate, women must be between the ages of 35 and 65, and live at least twenty-five miles away from a city of 12,500 or more, and have a chronic health condition.

Weinert explains the eligibility requirements. Women are more likely than men to join support groups. Very young women and very old women tend to have very different issues, so the age limits ensure some commonality among participants. The geographic requirement removes women who may have more easy access to other, nonvirtual, support groups. And the chronic condition qualifier is, of course, obvious.

Participation in the program is free. Women are, however, asked and, if need be, nudged to fully engage. Weinert estimates the program requires about four hours a week from each woman.

Another Voice, A Similar Story

Gerri Rouane echoes Sperandeo's appreciation for Women to Women.

Rouane, age 55, lives in Roundup, Montana, population some 3,000, fifty miles north of Billings. For years, she lived with the chronic pain of what she believed to be rheumatoid arthritis and treatments that did not work. Then, five years ago, she was finally diagnosed with fibromyalgia.

"I knew nothing about this condition," says Rouane. "[The doctor] gave me a pamphlet, and that was about it. The doctors tell you what you have, but they don't tell you how to deal with it."

"Once you're diagnosed with an illness that's going to be with you for the rest of your life, it humbles you. You feel like your body has become your enemy. I didn't know how to accept it and then how to deal with it."

Like Sperandeo, however, Rouane found out about Women to Women and signed on. And that, she says, changed her life.

"[The women] became my sisters," says Rouane. "I can't emphasize that enough. They became my family …. I came to love them for their strength, their hardiness ….To be in the company of very strong women who are living with illnesses that would defy that they're human because [the illnesses] are so bad."

The program also, she says, "opened a whole new world for me. It gave me the tools to be my own advocate. The tools to go online and figure out the medical terminology, or find a site especially for fibromyalgia, or ideas on how to manage my chronic pain."

Indeed, both women say that the program empowered them and, as a result, improved not only their emotional state but also their physical health. Not surprisingly, both women have encouraged others they know to apply.

Results

While Weinert and her team are pleased with the results so far, being researchers, they refrain from declaring victory.

"The intent of the study has never been to measure health utilization outcomes per se," says Weinert. "We're trying to change behaviors. … If a woman has better self-esteem, she may be more likely to [better manage her health]."

All Weinert will allow at this point is that "the results are going in the right direction. We're increasing support and reducing depression." But, she says, "Until we have statistically demonstrated results, we can't

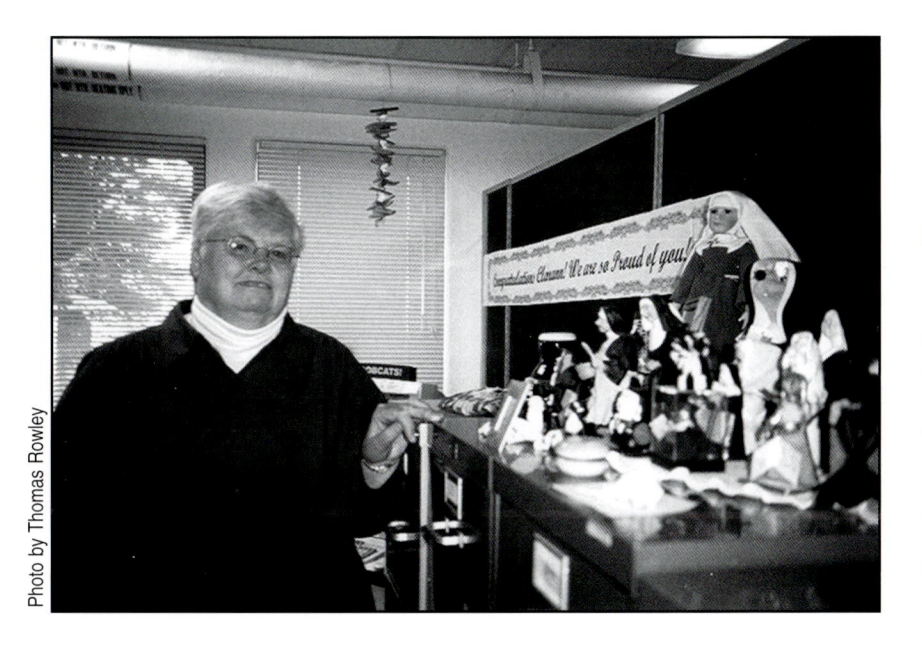

". . . the results are going in the right direction. We're increasing support and reducing depression."

Clarann Weinert

institutionalize it as a model. We have to illustrate that it will make a difference, before we can sell it."

There is no doubt, however, in the minds of Rouane and Sperandeo that the program makes a difference.

"You don't feel so helpless," says Rouane. "It gives you a life plan that you can work with."

Sperandeo says it even more forcefully, "It was my lifeline. It saved my life."

Notes:
The women interviewed for this story gave their permission to be included and reviewed the information prior to publication.

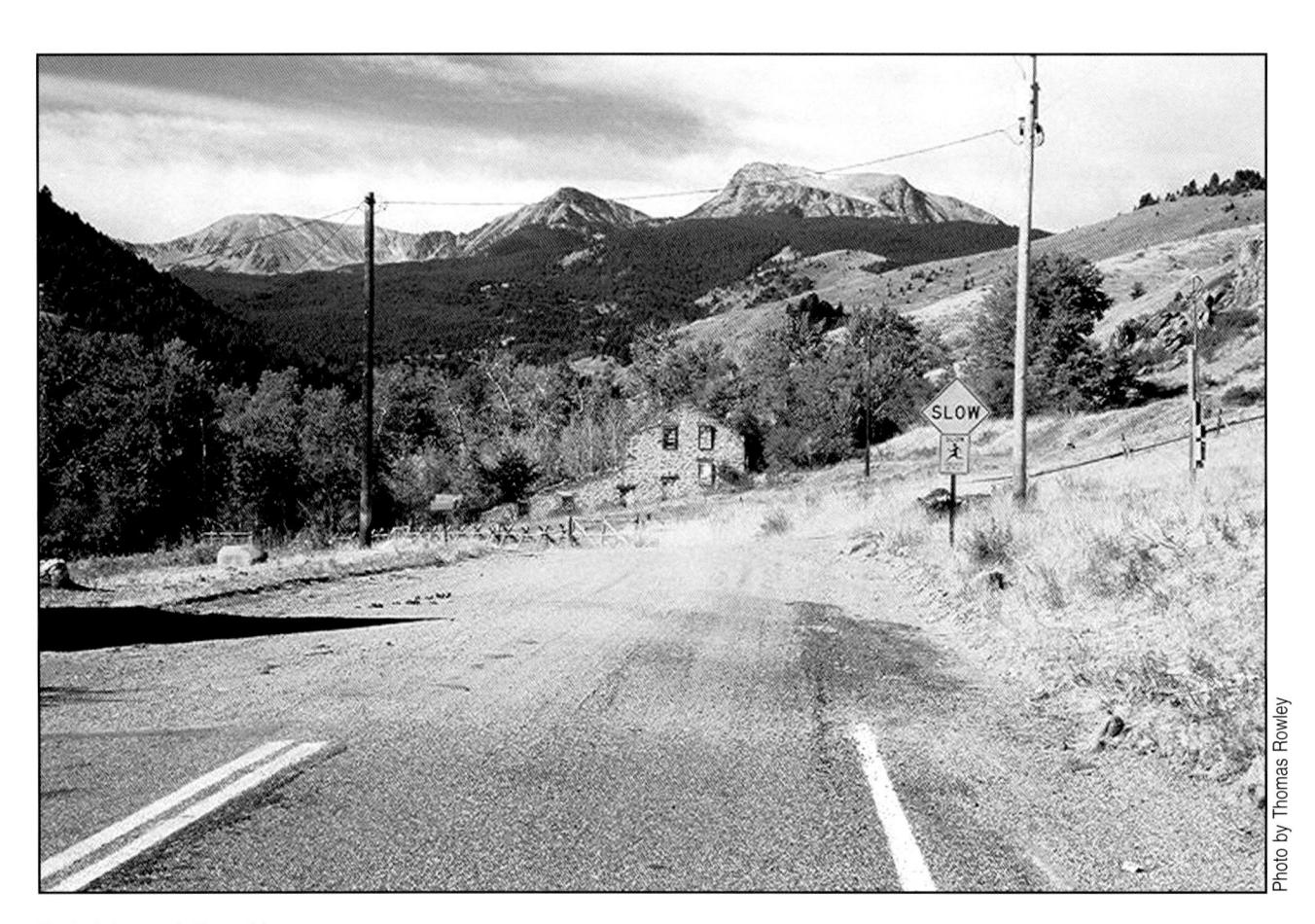

End of the road, Pony, Montana.

Photo by Thomas Rowley

Just the Facts

Purpose

Women to Women uses the Internet to link together in a virtual support network women who live in remote areas and have chronic medical conditions, evaluates the effectiveness of the process.

Target Population

The program is for women aged 35 to 65 with a chronic illness who live at least twenty-five miles from a population center of 12,500 or more.

Partners

Women to Women is a project of the Center for Research on Chronic Health Conditions in Rural Dwellers at the Montana State University-Bozeman, College of Nursing. Partners include the Burns Telecommunications Center at Montana State University-Bozeman. Funding comes from twelve different entities, including the Sisters of Charity Ministry Foundation and the National Institutes of Health/National Institute of Nursing Research (grant no. 5 ROI NR07908).

Budget

Annual costs are approximately $130,000, not including in-kind contributions.

Results

To date, 277 women have completed the program. Many report improvements in their self-esteem, emotional state, and overall health.

For more information, contact Clarann Weinert, Ph.D., Director, at cweinert@montana.edu.

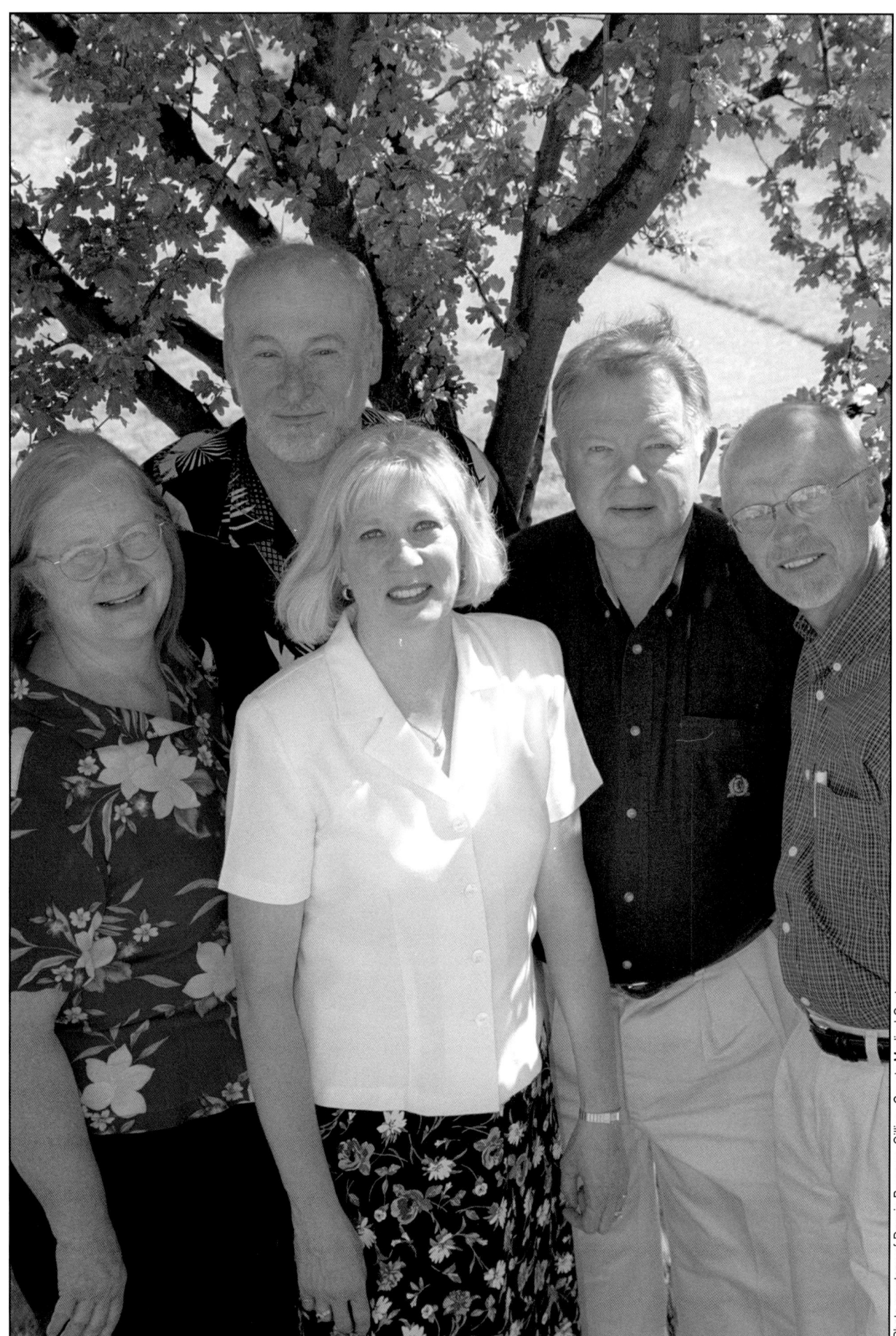

Photo courtesy of Dennis Bruneau, Gilliam County Medical Center

Providing (and Paying for) Frontier Care: Gilliam County Medical Center—Oregon

Few people, it's fair to say, happen upon Condon, Oregon. Indeed, just getting to this frontier town of 650 residents in the rolling hills of eastern Oregon takes some doing. Seventy-two miles of two-lane road from the interstate and the nearest town of any size makes for an hour and a half trip, in good weather.

Getting full-time health care to Condon also took some doing. Specifically, it took a vote, a tax increase, and a step into uncharted territory.

"We didn't have any health care and we're seventy-two miles away from a doctor or a hospital," says Condon's Bonnie Johnson. "It's not just a hop, skip, and jump to a big city. You see our winters. It wasn't a safe place to live without health care."

And yet that's what the people of the area—designated as both a Medically Underserved Area and a Health Professional Shortage Area—had been doing in one fashion or another for some time.

According to Johnson, the town had a clinic and had, in the past, had doctors and health practitioners, but the arrangements hadn't worked out.

"Because we just had one [provider] at a time, they'd burn out," says Johnson. "In a small town, if they don't answer their phone or aren't on call, people go to their house. People burn out quickly."

Built in the early 1950s, the clinic had been staffed by various providers over the years—some private, some with the National Health Service

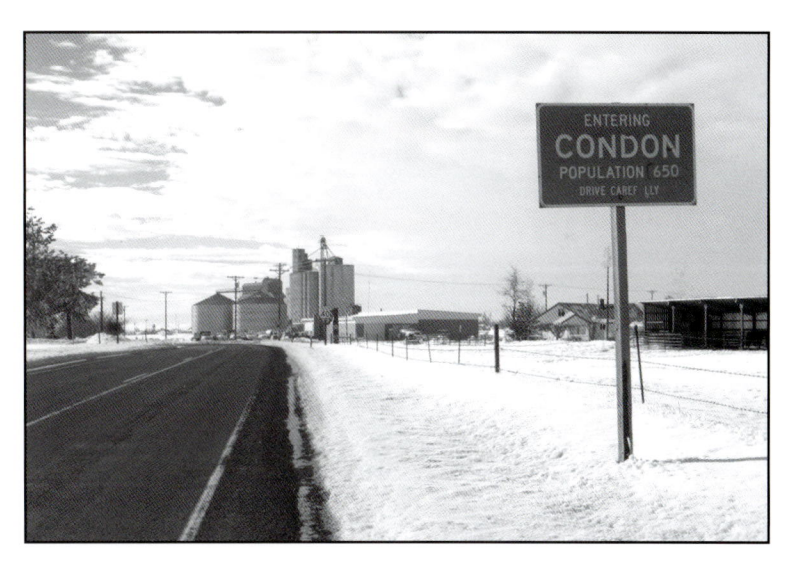

Photo opposite page: Staff of Gilliam County Medical Center (l to r) Karen Jones, David Jones, Cindy Hess, Bruce Carlson, M.D., and Dennis Bruneau.

Corps—until the late 1970s. Some of those providers retired; others could not make a full-time practice financially feasible; still others were hampered by laws preventing so-called mid-level practitioners from such things as prescribing medicines. By 1978, the sole provider at the clinic, and in the area, came just once a week, from 120 miles away.

Johnson and others decided they needed "to do something more permanent." With help from the Oregon State Office of Rural Health, they came up with the idea of creating a health care district to generate funds dedicated to health care. As with a school district or any other public district, boundaries are set and a tax is levied on property within those boundaries. A publicly elected board oversees the district. Creating such a district requires going to the public for a vote.

With help from the Oregon State Office of Rural Health, they came up with the idea of creating a health care district to generate funds dedicated to health care.

"By the time we got everything in order and went to the vote to fund the district," says Johnson, who served on the board in its first years, "it was like three or four to one. It was a huge landslide in favor."

The resulting tax bite—eighty-three cents per thousand—costs the average property owner about as much as a visit to the doctor.

That was 1980, and according to at least one researcher, the South Gilliam County Health District, as it came to be known, was the first primary care health district in the nation. Getting the district and property tax in place, however, is only half the story. The other half involves getting the providers in place.

The Program

With the funds from the tax in hand, the district board went looking for providers. The initial plan was to hire a physician assistant. (In 1979, the state legislature authorized physician assistants to work remotely from their supervising doctor and to prescribe medicines.)

"They called me and asked if I knew any PAs [physician assistants] interested in coming to Condon," says Dennis Bruneau, a physician assistant then on staff at the University of Washington. "I asked if they'd consider hiring two instead."

The reason: Bruneau had recently finished two and a half years as a physician assistant with the National Health Service Corps, serving as the sole health care provider in a remote village in Alaska.

"I'd burned out," he says.

Rather than running that risk again in Condon, Bruneau suggested to community leaders that they hire two providers to share the load. Having already lost providers to burnout, folks in Condon went along with the idea. Bruneau then approached Dave Jones, a colleague at the university; the two went out to Condon, interviewed, liked what they saw, and started looking for a doctor under whom they could practice. The search led them to Bruce Carlson, M.D., the doctor who had been traveling to serve at the clinic in Condon once a week. The three agreed to be a team, but one last hurdle had to be cleared.

Bruneau and Jones were both married to professional women, one a health professional, the other a manager. Because both women had careers and because both men would be taking pay cuts to come to Condon, they asked the board to take the "whole package." Bruneau and Jones would work as physician assistants, Karen Jones as a medical technician and coordinator of the volunteer ambulance service, and Cindy Hess (Bruneau's spouse) as office and finance manager. Again, the board agreed.

With the team assembled, the health district contracted with Carlson to run the clinic. Carlson, in turn, hired the two couples. In October 1980, Condon and the surrounding region got full-time 24/7 health care. Carlson comes every two weeks and is always available to the PAs for phone consults. Bruneau and Jones trade off covering nights and weekends. Karen Jones and Cindy Hess work 40 hours a week and then some.

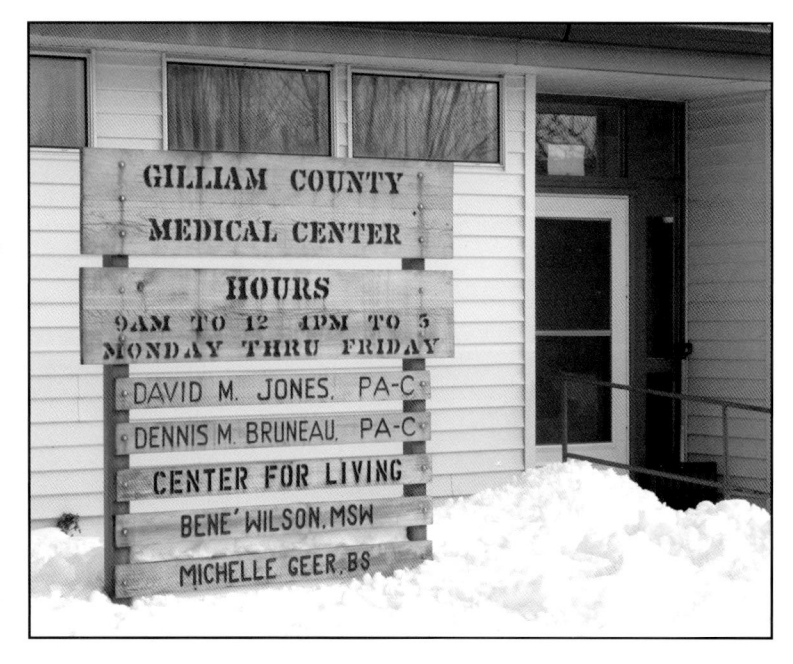

The clinic, Gilliam County Medical Center, is a private-public partnership. The district owns the building and the equipment, rents it to Carlson, and uses the tax money to subsidize Carlson. Currently, about $78,000, one-third of his budget, comes from the subsidy. Carlson does business as

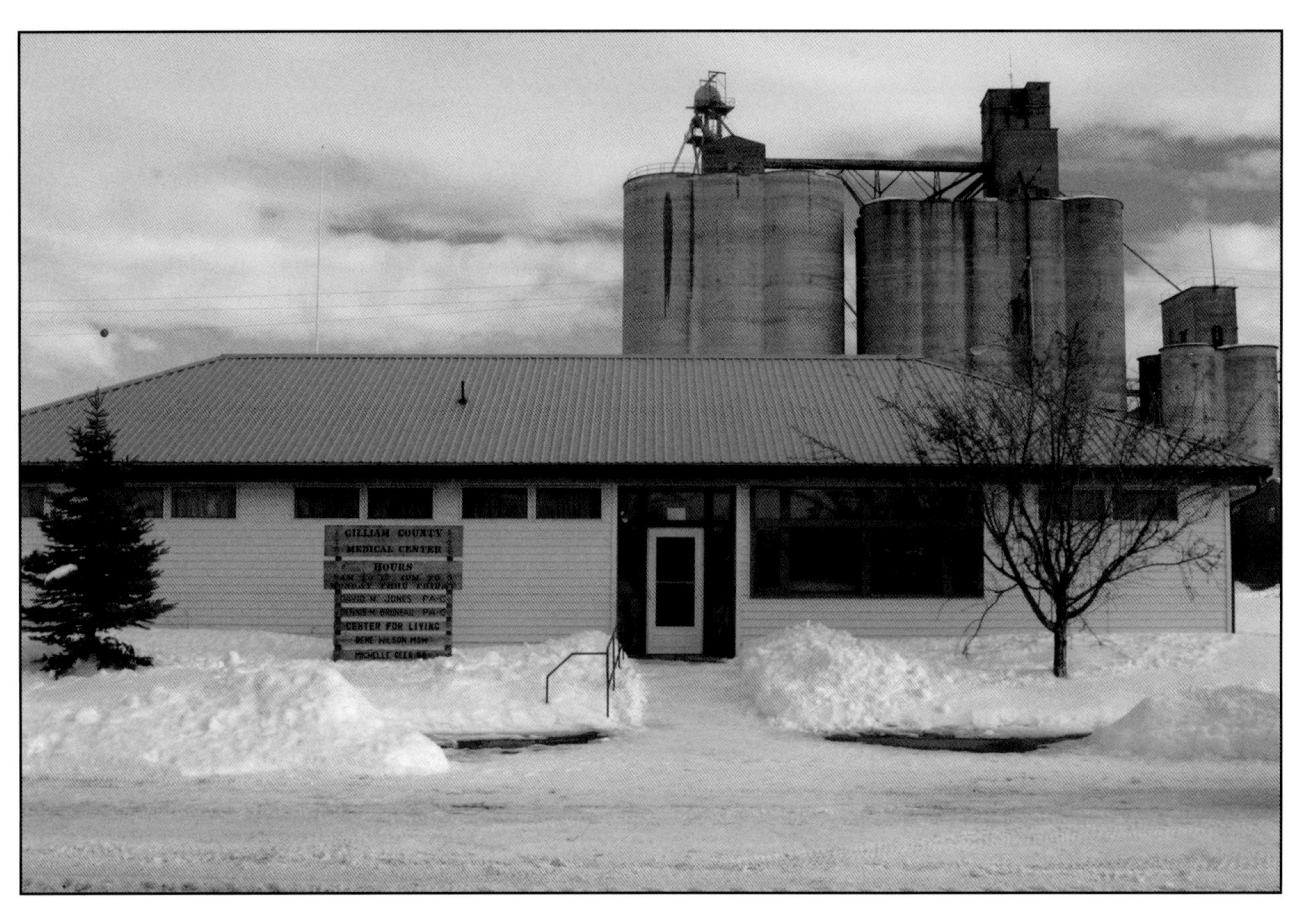

Gilliam County Medical Center.

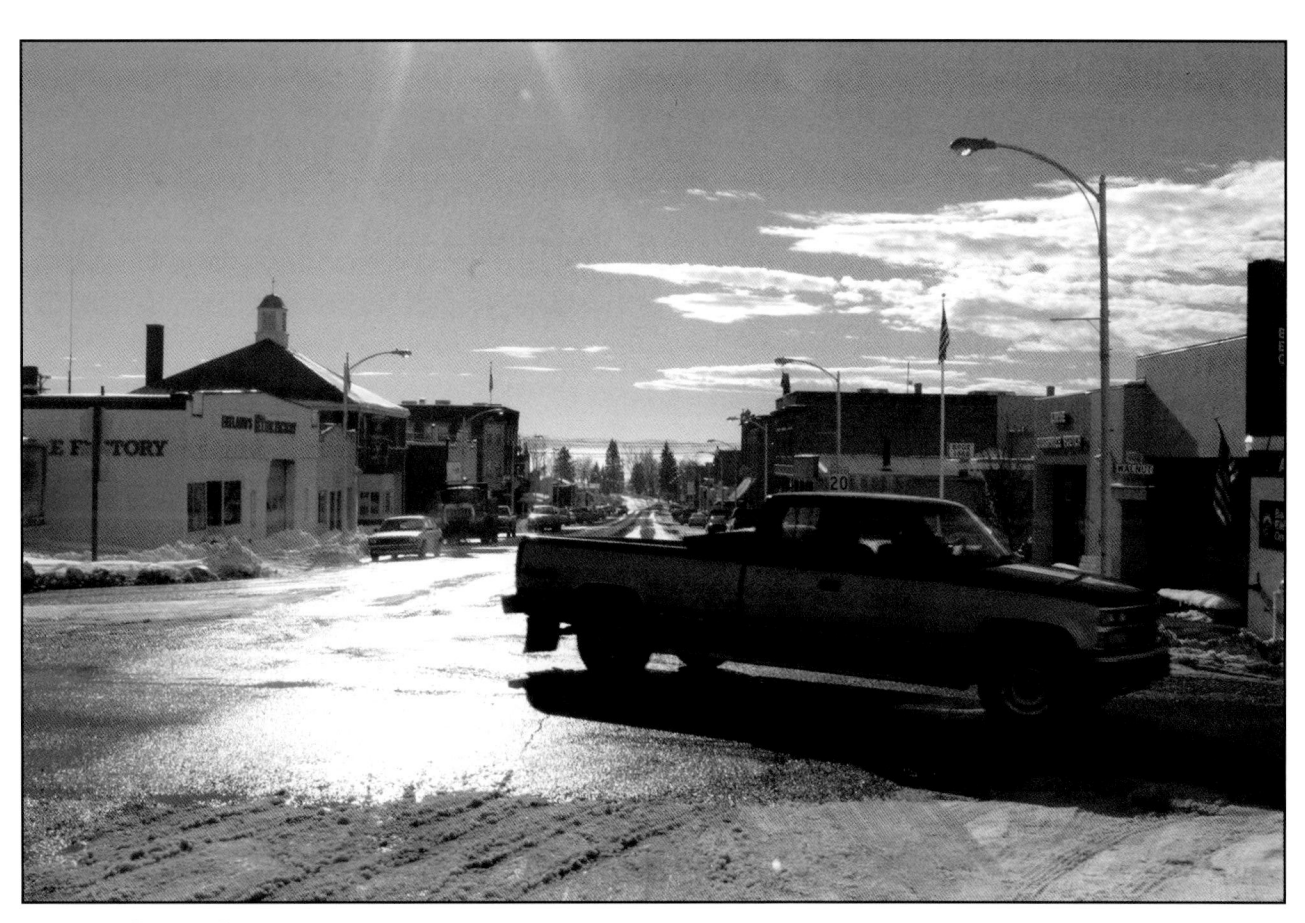

Downtown Condon, Oregon.

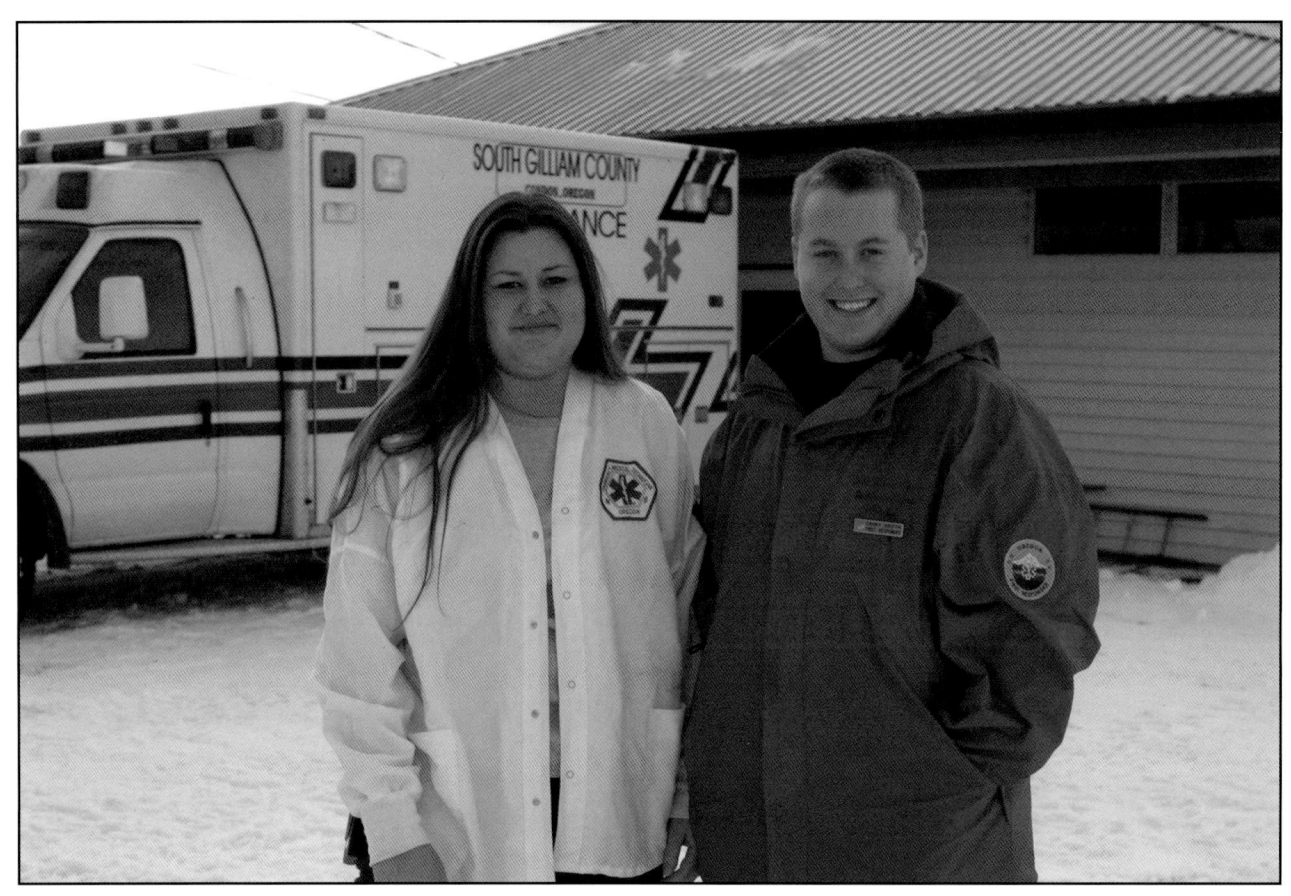

Denise Mann and Danny Hinton are high-school students trained as first responder EMTs.

a private-for-profit Rural Health Clinic, billing patients, insurance companies, and Medicare and Medicaid for services. At the end of each year, Carlson shares 25 percent of his profit with the district. Last year, he sent $9,000 back into the district's coffers. He also shares profits with the two PAs.

"We have the advantages of the public entity for the nonprofit stuff and then we have the advantages of the private-for-profit entity as far as wanting to be efficient," says Carlson. "A number of these things, the way they worked out was pure serendipity," he adds.

Indeed, all five agree that the success of the clinic hinges on two factors: the public subsidy and the skill and dedication of Carlson, Bruneau, Hess, Jones, and Jones.

"The patient volume would probably support one PA," says Carlson, "but the problem is with one PA we'd have provider burnout. We're successful because we have tax support. Economically, we could not do this without some sort of supplemental income."

Hess, who manages the finances, agrees. "Having the tax money makes the biggest difference. You know you're going to have dollars coming in every year."

And because each of the four handles a range of tasks, the clinic saves money.

"What kills frontier clinics like this is economics, not taking in enough revenue," says Bruneau. "The four of us are multi-discipline. Hiring a specialist for each is just not economically feasible. You can't be hiring an x-ray technician, a lab technician, a medical assistant, and a nurse. …It's just not economically feasible and practical."

As for dedication, the five exude it.

"This is what I was trained to do, primary care in a rural area," says Bruneau.

Of her husband, Karen Jones says, "He needed to do this kind of work."

Finally, there is Carlson, the man Dave Jones says is the perfect match for Condon. "He knows what it takes both medicine-wise and business-wise to keep a place like this going…he's committed to rural health."

All five agree that the success of the clinic hinges on two factors: the public subsidy and the skill and dedication of Carlson, Bruneau, Hess, Jones, and Jones.

> *"You're more involved with a lot of members of the community, because you're their doctor. That can be rewarding."*
>
> Bruce Carlson

He is indeed committed. Winner of the National Rural Health Association's 2001 Rural Health Practitioner of the Year Award, Carlson practices medicine in three different rural clinics. To do that, he travels 2,300 miles a month. The pace, he says, takes its toll. "Medicine is a demanding mistress." Nonetheless, he has no plans to retire (though he has left the clinic business to Hess in his will, to keep it going.)

"I'm having fun," says Carlson. "You go to the service station and you know the kid who's pumping your gas or you know his family. You go to the grocery store and you know the kid that's bagging groceries or [you know] his family. Maybe the checker at the grocery store, you delivered her last baby. You're more involved with a lot of members of the community, because you're their doctor. That can be rewarding."

Results

While the clinic's service area covers 1,100 square miles that are home to about 1,000 people, its yearly patient volume is approximately 3,500 visits, a higher than expected rate of capture.

"We have almost one and half times the number of visits one would expect," says Carlson.

That fact proclaims the clinic's success: people from outside the area prefer it over closer facilities.

The clinic, says Johnson, has "just worked absolutely perfectly for this community."

Just the Facts

Purpose

Gilliam County Medical Center is a Rural Health Clinic serving South Gilliam County, Oregon. Since 1980, it has provided medical care seven days a week, twenty-four hours a day in an area that previously had none. The next closest medical facility is seventy-two miles away.

Target Population

The center serves approximately 1,000 people living in an 1,100-square-mile area.

Partners

The center is a partnership of South Gilliam County Health District and Dr. Bruce Carlson.

Budget

Annual budget is $325,000 per year, 24 percent ($78,000 last year) of which comes as subsidy from the health district.

Results

The clinic sees approximately 3,500 patient visits per year.

For more information, contact Cindy Hess, Office Manager, Gilliam County Medical Center, at chess@oregonvos.net.

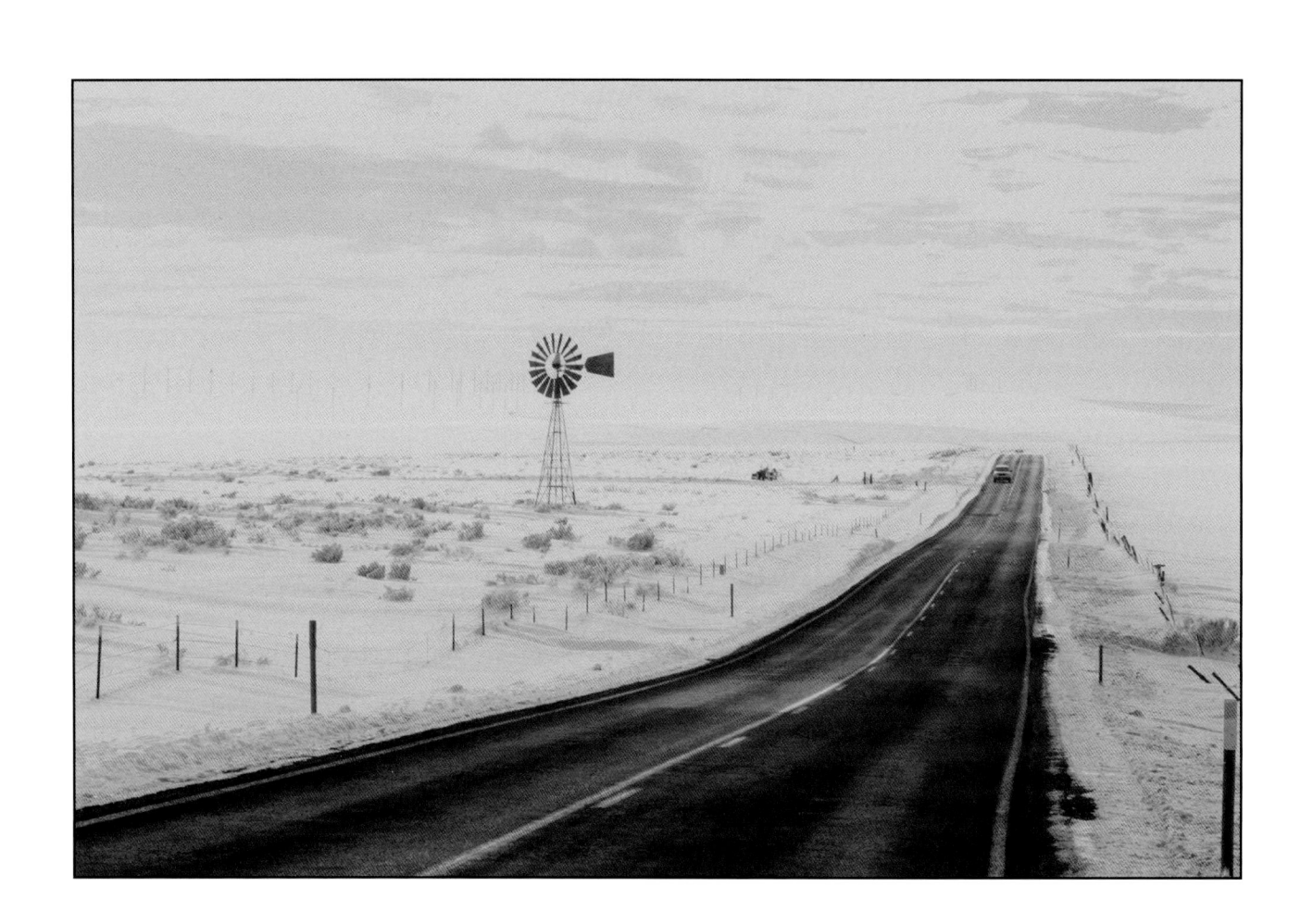

Nursing by Phone:
Visiting Nurses of Aroostook—Maine

Aroostook County, Maine's northern-most county, spreads for 6,672 square miles—an area bigger than Connecticut and Rhode Island combined. And while it accounts for 22 percent of the state's land, the county is home to but 6 percent of Maine's population. To say it's "remote" is something of an understatement. To reach that 6 percent with health care is something of a challenge.

The Visiting Nurses of Aroostook (VNA), however, are helping meet that challenge in person and, more recently, over the phone. This private, not-for-profit organization with a staff of approximately fifty nurses provides in-home care to the people of Aroostook County, as well as the northern portions of Penobscot and Washington Counties, where there are few providers to cover patients' needs.

Part of the Aroostook Home Care Agency, VNA has been sending nurses out into the surrounding country since 1989. In 1999, it increased its capacity by launching the Northeast Maine Telemedicine NetWork, a high-tech program that allows nurses to monitor a patient's status via a videophone. Funding came from a $450,000 grant made by the Robert Wood Johnson Foundation.

The program provides patients with telemedicine units for their homes. The units simply plug into the phone line (plain old telephone service) and an electrical outlet, yet provide two-way live video between patient and nurse. In addition, the units are fitted with such things as blood pressure cuffs, stethoscopes, scales, glucometers, and pulse oximeters, depending on a patient's need, to aid the nurse in monitoring a patient's condition. When the nurse calls, the patient picks up the phone, flips some switches, and the check-up begins.

Nurses from VNA still must travel out to patients for in-person visits, but with the new technology, fewer of those visits are needed. And by cutting down on time spent driving from house to house, the nurses can actually see their patients more often, project directors say.

According to Julie Codrey, R.N., Telemedicine Coordinator, VNA served more than 100 clients last year with the technology and made more than 500 televisits. The technology, she said, saved the agency $46,000 last year.

Most of VNA's patients are elderly. Some, in fact, are in hospice. Others, however, are just starting out in life. Codrey recalls using the technology in reverse to enable a busy farmer to "visit" his premature baby girl every night from home, while the infant stayed in the neonatal care unit, hours away.

In a remote area like northern Maine, says Codrey, it's often telemedicine or else a very long trip.

For more information, contact Julie Codrey, Telemedicine Coordinator, at (207) 532-9261.

Afterword

Arlington, Virginia–Writing about rural America while sitting three subway stops from downtown Washington, D.C., is, I admit, somewhat ironic. To some, it may be downright presumptuous. I confess: I am not a rural person—despite spending the last 16 years focusing on rural issues, not to mention growing up with a cow pasture for a backyard (in what I later learned was a metropolitan county).

Still, my location offers two distinct advantages. First, it affords me the relative objectivity of an interested, yet outside, observer. That, in turn, allows me—if only occasionally—to be heard when other, more knowledgeable, voices might be dismissed, however wrongly, for being "swayed by self interest."

Second, it puts me near the federal action that so greatly affects what happens in and to rural America. The meetings, briefings, and hearings held by congressional committees, governmental agencies, and associations of every stripe yield great fodder for writing.

Neither advantage, however, is without cost. One reduces far too much of my experience with rural people and places to statistics in a table, words on a page, and an occasional voice on the phone. The other often leaves me despairing of real progress, let alone solutions.

The opportunity then to get out into the countryside and meet people in need and people filling that need was both edifying and uplifting. It increased my understanding of the issues and it raised my hopes for the future. The needs of rural America are great; the responses of her people are greater. By seeing that firsthand, by sitting with people shedding tears of pain and those shedding tears of gratitude, I learned more than can be gotten from stacks of reports or months of meetings and lost whatever objectivity I may have had.

I hope that in the pages of this book readers sense enough of that pain and gratitude to inspire them to continue or to start anew their own efforts at providing care wherever they are, whatever tools are at hand, no matter the obstacles that lay before them. For while much good has been done, much more remains to be done. Speaking, I hope, for us all, Sister Bernadette Kenny, a nurse practitioner and medical missionary in southern Appalachia, sums it up, "I wish I had started earlier and that it didn't take so long."

In *The Healer's Calling*, physician and Franciscan friar Daniel P. Sulmasy writes:

> *Magic is a zap from the sky, but healing is a deeply human process. Magic is impersonal, but healing involves intimacy and relationships.*

The efforts chronicled here are not magic. There are no hidden tricks, nothing which cannot be replicated. They are healing efforts. Each one—whatever its innovation—is a deeply human process involving intimacy and relationships, delivering not just health care, but care…and hope.

And in today's world, that may be the most important innovation of all.

Tom Rowley

Acknowledgments

Working on this book gave Brent Miller and me the distinct privilege of going to some of this nation's most beautiful places, meeting some of its friendliest people, and capturing in words and photos some of its most innovative rural health efforts. We are extremely grateful to all who made that possible.

Obviously, this collection of stories would not exist without the people who created the stories—the men and women in rural America who dedicate their lives to improving the lives of others. We thank them for their efforts on behalf of their neighbors and for sharing those efforts with us. We also thank those on the receiving end of care for sharing their stories and in several cases welcoming us into their homes.

We are deeply indebted to Eli Briggs and Alan Morgan at the National Rural Health Association, and Marcia Brand, Tom Morris and Jennifer Riggle at HRSA's Office of Rural Health Policy for the opportunity (and funding) to work on the project and for their thoughtful guidance throughout. Special thanks go to Jennifer for coming up with the idea for the book.

Choosing projects to include in these pages was no easy task. Suggestions came from all over the country, all good. Space, however, was limited. Therefore, we are grateful for the assistance of an advisory panel in helping select which projects to include and in shaping the outline of the book. Members of that panel were Denise Denton of the Colorado Rural Health Center; Jeff Hanson of the New England Rural Health Roundtable; Glen Massengale of Monticello, Kentucky; Kristy Nichols of the Louisiana Office of Rural Health, and Debra Phillips of Southern Illinois University and Quincy Family Practice. Carol Miller of the Frontier Education Center, Evan Mayfield and Jerry Coopey of HRSA's Office of Rural Health Policy, and Kathy Williams of the Iowa Office of Rural Health also kindly helped. None, of course, are responsible for any shortcomings of the book.

Scheduling our visits, seeing the things we needed to see, and interviewing the people we needed to interview would have been impossible without the generous and able assistance of Vickie Kasprzyk in California, LaJuan Scott in Texas, Cindy Hess in Oregon, Lynn Niewohner in Illinois, Chris Palombo and Kayla West in Michigan, Fran Feltner and David Gross in Kentucky, Carolyn Sliger in Tennessee, Clarann Weinert and Dave Young in Montana, Gina Radechel and Steve Simonin in Iowa, and Russ Sword and Pam Ferguson in Arkansas. Many thanks also to Shirley Cudney for a wonderful drive across Montana, to Wade Hill for an incredible trout-filled side trip down Montana's Missouri River, and to Sabrina Feltner and Anna Sloan for letting us tag along as they made their rounds in Kentucky.

On the readability front, thanks to Becky Flynt for telling me what did and didn't make sense in early drafts and to Ann Donaldson for editing the final manuscript.

Last but not least, thanks to Maria, Jake, and Michael, and Lin for holding down the respective forts while Brent and I crisscrossed the countryside.

We hope that all parties, in some small way, think it was worth it. We do.

National Rural Health Association

The National Rural Health Association is a member-driven national organization whose mission is to improve the health of rural Americans and populations through appropriate and equitable health care services as well as to assist its members in providing leadership on rural issues through advocacy, communications, education, and research. To accomplish this, the association espouses the following values that express the association's concern not only with the provision of health care services, but with the level of health and well-being that those services establish for rural areas and their residents.

- All Americans are entitled to an equitable level of health and well-being established through health care services regardless of geographic locale, gender, ethnic or racial background, or economic ability or status.

- Access to primary and preventive health care services should be available locally to rural residents to achieve the goal of preventing illness whenever possible.

- An overarching goal of the association is to foster service partnerships among health care providers and facilities, rather than focusing on the disciplines.

- The association recognizes the value that each member brings to the improvement of rural health care services and values the multicultural diversity of its membership. Additionally, the association realizes the broader scope of solutions and opportunities that may be achieved through the grassroots efforts of this membership.

- The association recognizes that collegiality and partnerships with and among other associations may serve to enhance or increase rural health accomplishments.

- The association believes local residents should be involved in determining the health care needed and provided in their community.

- The association values and strives to achieve its role in helping members provide the best possible health care services by offering continuing education and information on rural health related issues, policy and research.

The association values its role in improving rural health care services and thereby positively affecting the public health of rural people and populations. Through the improvement of its members, other organizations, and government entities, assistance is provided in achieving a more positive health care environment and maximum health status for all rural Americans. To this end, the association strives to be a proactive and positive force in its efforts toward providing the best rural health care possible.

For more information, see www.nrharural.org.

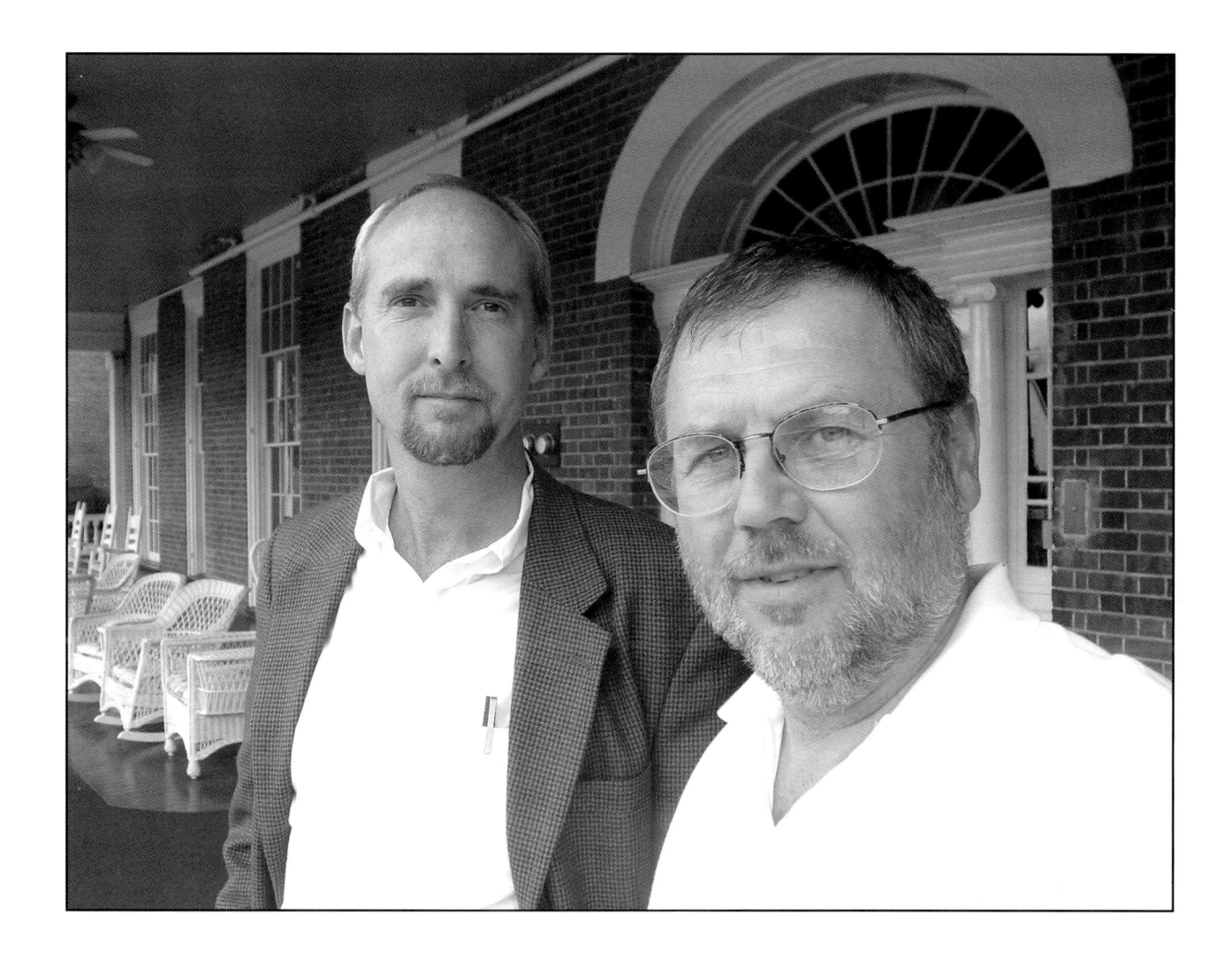

Tom Rowley is a syndicated columnist, editor of *The Rural Monitor*, and a fellow at the Rural Policy Research Institute. Most of his work focuses on rural people, places, and the issues facing them.

Past positions include stints with the TVA Rural Studies Program at the University of Kentucky, *Forum for Applied Research and Public Policy*, and the U.S. Department of Agriculture's Economic Research Service. At USDA, he also worked with the National Rural Development Partnership, the National Commission on Agriculture and Rural Development Policy, the President's Council on Sustainable Development, the Office of Management and Budget, and the Organization for Economic Cooperation and Development.

He lives with his family outside Washington, DC.

D. Brent Miller is a writer and photographer who has focused on small towns and rural issues since 1985. He is a former professor of journalism and photojournalism, Loras College, Dubuque, Iowa, and has worked for daily and weekly newspapers in his native Illinois.

He served as the newsletter editor for the National Rural Development Partnership, and was a governing board member of the Indiana Rural Development Council, serving as their chair for the Rural Arts and Culture Task Force.

He holds a B.A. in Applied Christian Studies from Trinity College, Deerfield, Illinois, and an M.A. in Journalism and M.A. in Communication Studies from Northern Illinois University, DeKalb, Illinois.

Brent and his wife reside in Granger, Indiana. More of Brent's photography can be seen at www.DBrent.com.